WITHOUT CONSENT

WITHOUT CONSENT

SHEILA O CONNOR

WITHDRAWN

POOLBEG

Published 2010
by Poolbeg Books Ltd
123 Grange Hill, Baldoyle,
Dublin 13, Ireland
Email: poolbeg@poolbeg.com

1 3 5 7 9 10 8 6 4 2

A catalogue record for this book is available from the British Library.

ISBN 978-1-84223-407-5

Typeset by Patricia Hope in Sabon 11/15
Printed by Litografia Rosés S.A., Spain

www.poolbeg.com

About the Author

Sheila O Connor is a founding member of Patient Focus, a charity dedicated to promoting dignity in health care. She has worked as a patient advocate for fourteen years. She coordinated support for women and families affected by the Neary scandal and was actively involved in their campaign for justice.

I would like to dedicate this book to Baby Eileen, Baby Hannah, Baby James and Baby Sean.

Contents

Prologue

Brief History of a Scandal

This is the story of women who trusted a hospital and a doctor. The hospital is Our Lady of Lourdes Hospital, Drogheda, County Louth, a revered institution in the town and surrounding areas.

Young women went in through its doors to welcome the joyful arrival of a new baby and returned home to grieve the loss of their womb, future children and grandchildren. Other women entered its gynaecology unit with minor and benign conditions and emerged profoundly damaged. This damage was horrifically described by a Harley Street doctor as "castration".

It was in this hospital that these women encountered Michael Neary, a doctor feared and admired in equal measure.

The Town and the Hospital
Drogheda is a middle-sized Irish town off the motorway between two large cities, Dublin and Belfast. Its lush agricultural hinterland is renowned worldwide for the Stone Age burial chambers, royal and monastic settlements and

1

ecclesiastical sites dotted throughout the Boyne valley, like apples on a richly laden bough. The town itself is famous for the deeds of two men named Oliver – Oliver Cromwell and Saint Oliver Plunkett. Cromwell's army stormed the town and massacred large numbers of its people in the mid-seventeenth century. It is famous too as a place of pilgrimage. One of its churches houses the severed head of Saint Oliver Plunkett, a Catholic shrine to a patriot bishop executed by the English. Many Irish school children are brought by their teachers to visit Drogheda. On school outings, they can be seen climbing the steps of St Peter's Church to view the saint's head, as well as queuing to visit the other historic and prehistoric sites in the region.

Drogheda's maternity hospital was established by the Medical Missionaries of Mary under its founder, Mother Mary Martin. It was officially opened on 8 December 1939. This is the Roman Catholic holy day that celebrates the belief that Mary, the virgin mother of Jesus, was conceived without original sin and is therefore most perfect.

It was here that many women from the north-eastern region of Ireland came to have their babies, believing that they were receiving the best of care, both for themselves and for their babies.

At first the Lourdes was purely a maternity hospital which looked after the mothers of Drogheda and surrounding areas. It also trained doctors and nurses for the African missions. Its Catholic ethos prohibited all forms of artificial contraception. Information on artificial measures was not allowed, even if pregnancy was dangerous. Sterilisation for contraceptive purposes was not permitted. But *indirect* sterilisation, primarily for medical reasons, was allowed. In

Catholic hospitals this usually involved the isolation of the "diseased organ" by removing the womb. Tubal ligation – the tying of the fallopian tube to prevent fertilisation – was unacceptable.

Throughout its history, the structure of the maternity hospital was rigidly hierarchical and authoritarian, with either the consultants or the management of the Medical Missionaries occupying the pivotal position. Midwives were very much at the bottom of the professional ladder. They clearly knew their place, which was to do as they were told and ask no questions, in a profoundly paternalistic environment. Their powerlessness in this unit was second only to the powerlessness of the women who trusted the unit and its staff to deliver their babies and keep them safe. There was no avenue for either midwife or patient to address queries or concerns at the unit and if they did arise, they were quickly snuffed out.

The maternity hospital, throughout its history, operated as a separate institution, even when a general hospital was built about 300 metres away.

Michael Neary was Untouchable

It was here that Michael Neary was appointed as a consultant obstetrician/gynaecologist in 1974, when he was thirty-one years of age. He had qualified as a doctor from University College Galway in 1965 and became a Fellow of the Royal College of Obstetricians and Gynaecologists in 1972. He obtained intern training in Galway and he subsequently was Senior House Officer in Withington Teaching Hospital in Manchester.

He had difficulty getting another job after this. One of

his consultants wouldn't allow him to work in theatre and gave him a bad reference. This conflict arose, he told the Lourdes Hospital Inquiry, because of his ethical opposition to tubal ligation and termination. This is odd, given his subsequent history in Drogheda.

At any rate he changed his referee and, as a result, he got a post as Registrar in Obstetrics and Gynaecology in St Mary's Hospital, Portsmouth. He was there from November 1968 to January 1971. At that time, on the recommendation of his old Galway teacher, he went to Hammersmith Hospital as Senior Registrar, where he worked under a doctor with strong Catholic beliefs. He stayed there until April 1974. From April 1974 to December 1998 he practised in the Lourdes Hospital.

He fitted in quickly, due to his apparent easy charm, hard-working ethos and high opinion of his own professional abilities. He copper-fastened his rapidly growing reputation as a safe pair of hands and committed doctor by his heroic stories of women saved from imminent death at childbirth by his surgical skills. He was not shy in telling these women and their families how he rescued them from death by removing their wombs, often at the birth of their first or second baby (caesarean hysterectomy).

As Neary grew in reputation, the other two obstetricians seemed happy to leave much in the safe hands of this new hard-working, apparently talented doctor. At any rate, they didn't interfere in each other's practice or comment in particular on the care of private patients.

Neary's rapid resort to caesarean hysterectomy became a characteristic of his practice at the Lourdes. The figures were there for all to see. But people from outside the unit rarely visited, let alone questioned its practices. During his time at the Lourdes, Dr Neary was also engaged in damaging gynaecological surgery. As far back as the late 1970s, he began his mutilating practice of removing both ovaries from a number of young women, many of them with no children. They were immediately catapulted into an early menopause and denied the right to have children. After this, many viewed themselves as having the body of an old woman rather than someone in their twenties, thirties or forties. Neary justified the surgery by saying they had serious disease when in fact their conditions were benign, self-limiting or treatable in other ways. Neary's gynaecological surgery took place in the gynaecology unit in the main hospital and not in the maternity unit, which was concerned with the delivery of babies. No one noticed it, or if they did they kept their mouths tightly shut.

Attempts to Tell

Isolation, dogma, hierarchical structure and the powerlessness of women allowed Neary's activities to go largely, though not completely, unchallenged during his twenty-four-year tenure at the hospital. For the very few who did raise a query, unravelling the truth about Neary was akin to attempting to untie tangled knots from knitting wool. The more one tried, the tighter and more twisted the knots became. In the end Neary became untouchable and women patients were abandoned to their fate.

At least, that is how it appears from Judge Maureen Harding Clark's account of the efforts to tell by a patient, the matron and by a nurse tutor in the late 1970s and early 1980s. Judge Harding Clark believes that if due attention had been paid to these attempts, many women could have been saved from injury by means of unnecessary caesarean hysterectomy at least. If the institution and doctor had not been put before the patients, many women would have been saved.

Majella, one of the patients, complained to a solicitor about Dr Neary in 1980. At the age of twenty-five, she suffered the loss of her womb at the birth of her second baby. She sought legal advice and was reluctantly persuaded that caesarean hysterectomy was carried out by Dr Neary only in cases of severe haemorrhage. She felt betrayed by her legal advisor at the time, as well as by the doctor she questioned. It was very difficult for a damaged patient to sue in the early 1980s, particularly when not supported in her attempt by her solicitor. She felt the system was very much stacked against her, but she wanted to have a go nonetheless. Irish doctors, she was told, would not give evidence against each other. She could lose her house if she lost. She was in a David versus Goliath contest and was very unlikely to win against the might of the medical profession. At any rate, her brave attempt was unsuccessful.

It is interesting to note too that she was first told of her hysterectomy after caesarean section at her post-natal check up with Dr Neary. She was very distressed and angry at his failure to tell her while she was an in-patient. She was a private patient but she was in a public ward after her surgery. She now believes that is why neither she nor her husband, who visited every day and often encountered Dr Neary during visiting hours, were not told while she was in the hospital.

The matron of the maternity unit called a meeting of the consultants to draw attention to Neary's high caesarean hysterectomy rate in 1978/9. At the meeting, one of the consultants commented that there were no maternal deaths.

Dr Neary said the hysterectomies were indirect sterilisations. The matron felt that Dr Neary himself deflected attention from her concerns by wrongly accusing a junior doctor at the unit of secretly carrying out tubal ligations. She also felt he tried to blame her for not noticing these forbidden procedures. The matron's attempt failed. She was bruised by this and afterwards felt Dr Neary treated her with contempt.

Coincidentally another attempt to untangle matters was also taking place at this time. A temporary midwifery tutor, who was also a Medical Missionary nun, was very worried about two caesarean hysterectomies carried out in August 1978 by Dr Neary. She believed the hysterectomies were not medically necessary. Whether her concerns were for "unethical" sterilisations, forbidden by the Church, or for the patients, or both, we don't know. But she tried to follow them up. Secretarial staff would not give her access to patient files to check if there were more such operations. She talked to the Cardinal, a senior member of the Catholic hierarchy, at the time about her worries. He told her this was a matter for the doctors. Judge Harding Clark tells us that these patient notes are missing.

Strangely, her action in discussing the matter outside the unit was considered disloyalty and she felt criticised by the matron. She left the hospital in late 1980, thinking the hysterectomies had stopped.

After this, Neary continued on unchecked. In the mid-1980s he went on a "binge", performing sixteen caesarean hysterectomies during 1985 and 1986. The fact that one of these women was the wife of a doctor having her first baby had the effect of quietening any anxieties that still remained about Neary.

Reading Judge Harding Clark's report gives the impression that a mere raised eyebrow or curl of the lip by management or consultants usually managed to stifle what queries arose. When this wasn't enough, comments about tubal ligation, maternal death and the duty of loyalty to the institution itself was sufficient to end questioning. Michael Neary continued his unusual obstetric practices unhindered. And no one seems to have noticed his strange gynaecological practices.

A New Unit
Meanwhile, by 1990 the new maternity unit was opened and it was no longer physically separate from the general hospital. Facilities for women improved immensely, but the old ethos, structures and working practices continued. So too did Michael Neary's practice of caesarean hysterectomy. Still there was no avenue to raise a concern. Not that it was needed, as most women believed the story about the danger to their life and prayed for the wonderful doctor who had assisted them.

Not all the women were happy, though. During the 1990s, a small number of women complained of other matters, unrelated to caesarean hysterectomy. When one woman requested her files after the scandal broke in 1998, her letter of complaint about Neary was not in her file. It had disappeared, as if she had never sent it.

Meanwhile Neary was operating away and the numbers of caesarean hysterectomies he performed were steadily growing. Between 1991 and 1993, he performed twenty. By 1996 the number had reached ten for the year, with six of them taking place in January. Still no one shouted stop.

The matron, however, continued to whisper her anxieties

and tried to tease Neary's knot of control open. She tried to raise the issue, tentatively now as she had been burned by her past efforts and was afraid of Neary. She queried the section rate in the hope that it would draw attention to the caesarean hysterectomy rate. Meetings were called but Dr Neary either failed to attend these meetings or left them in anger. Meanwhile young woman after young woman entered the hospital to welcome a new baby and often returned home grieving the loss of her womb and recovering from serious surgery. But the hierarchy remained undisturbed.

In 1996 a midwife at the hospital, Valerie Neary (no relation to Dr Michael Neary), suffered a horrific trauma while delivering her baby. Michael Neary removed her womb, despite her protests. This naturally caused much hurt at the unit and also raised questions about the practices of the doctor once again. Following this, a close friend of Valerie's asked the matron for help. The matron went with the Labour Ward Superintendent to make inquiries of the theatre staff and the anaesthetist who were there. They had no concerns about the need for the operation. The anaesthetist noted heavy bleeding and the midwives present remembered Neary saying Valerie had a defect in her uterus because of a drug taken by her mother. Clearly, once again matters were rationalised in favour of the doctor.

Some New Blood

A new Director of Nursing was appointed at the general hospital in 1996 and in May 1997 the North Eastern Health Board (NEHB) took over management and ownership of the hospital. This disappointed Michael Neary and Michael Shine who, in conjunction with others, wished to buy the hospital and continue to run it as a private concern. The Lourdes was now a public, state-run hospital in the care of lay people.

Some new midwives were recruited from outside the hospital too. They brought new knowledge, ideas and attitudes with them. Eventually, the new influx of fresh blood would upset the blind loyalty within the unit, as well as the long-established power of Michael Neary. In the end, it was an outsider, "Ann", a midwife who trained in the Royal Victoria Hospital, Belfast, who told the terrible story and finally unravelled the terrible truth about Neary and the Lourdes.

Of Ann, Judge Harding Clark says, "If it were in the power of the Inquiry to make an award of bravery to any person, it would be to the midwife who we shall call Ann." (Lourdes Hospital Inquiry, p. 188.)

Ann joined the unit in September 1997. The subservient role played by midwives in the unit was not Ann's way. She was concerned by the culture of intense loyalty to obstetricians, the lack of continuity of patient care and the absence of patient advocacy in the unit. It did not put women and their babies at the centre of care, she thought. Their interests were subordinated to that of Neary and the unit.

In theatre, she instantly questioned why she should "fetch the hysterectomy clamps" when requested to do so by Michael Neary and immediately made known her concerns about the ensuing hysterectomy. Her colleagues either did not wish to hear this criticism or found flaws with it. She, unlike them, did not admire Dr Neary. She was appalled that he routinely scarred women by his midline cuts at caesarean section. She was appalled that he carried out episiotomies routinely on women who had already had children. She was appalled that he placed women on their back with their legs in stirrups to deliver. But there was no forum for Ann to express her concerns about unacceptable care of the women having babies.

Ann became especially upset when she found out that hysterectomy was performed regularly and on some very young women. Her colleagues told her she had no evidence, so she took to documenting what she saw in theatre. She nagged her colleagues constantly and was beginning to see some shift in opinion. They told her there was nothing a midwife could do unless a patient complained. They told her consultants were clinically independent and could not be queried on their procedures. In particular, they told her one could not interfere with the treatment of private patients.

But by October 1998, the large numbers of young mothers having hysterectomies began to worry some other midwives too. The newer ones came from other hospitals where a wide range of family planning services existed. The older ones too were becoming seriously alarmed about Dr Neary's hysterectomy rate.

In early October 1998, "Ciara", a midwife trained in a large Dublin hospital, raised the issue of caesarean hysterectomy with a visiting professor from the midwifery school at Trinity College Dublin. During a discussion on assertiveness, Ciara told the professor, "We seem to have a lot of them here", meaning caesarean hysterectomy. Ciara's senior colleagues stayed silent; some even supported Dr Neary and said they saw no problem.

The Trinity professor was shocked, but her offer of help was turned down with a promise by the midwives that they would sort it out. However, the wind was taken out of Ciara's sails by this, and what happened next suggested that

11

history might be about to repeat itself almost twenty years later: the new Assistant Matron of the unit greatly admired Neary and Ciara was told off for being unprofessional, just as the midwifery tutor had been in 1980.

But then a very terrible thing happened. In early October, Niamh, a twenty-year-old patient, had a caesarean hysterectomy eighteen minutes after her first baby was born. "Dara", a midwifery tutor and practice nurse at the unit, heard about Niamh's hysterectomy in mid-October, during a lecture on postpartum haemorrhage she was giving to final-year students. The student thought Niamh's hysterectomy was appropriate. Initially, Dara didn't believe it had happened and felt the student must be mistaken. But she nevertheless decided to follow it up, only to discover that the student was right. She discussed it with Ann, Ciara and "Elaine", other midwives, all trained outside the Lourdes.

By now they had deep concerns. Something had to be done. One of them showed Dara where to find the maternity theatre register so she could check the number of cases of caesarean hysterectomy for 1998. She counted twelve or thirteen. Dara then told the Director of Nursing, Mary Duff, what she had discovered.

Ann decided to tell Gary Byrne, the Health Board's solicitor, about Dr Neary's caesarean hysterectomy rate. She and another midwife, "Brigid", had a prearranged meeting with him to discuss another problem on 22 October 1998.

At this meeting, Ann asked him if clinical independence went so far that questions could not be asked about serious concerns. The solicitor was disturbed at what she told him about Dr Neary. He contacted senior management shortly afterwards and the wheels of change were in motion.

Meanwhile, as Ann was telling the solicitor, Neary was doing another hysterectomy back at the hospital, this time on a woman who was thirty-three weeks pregnant. Ciara was involved in her care. She told the new Assistant Matron about this hysterectomy. She went to her office with the patient's chart. She brought Niamh's chart too. She was not even invited to sit down. She was told the patient was high-risk and generally dismissed. She did not believe Ciara that other maternity units did not have the same rate of hysterectomy.

By the next day, 23 October, the Director of Nursing, Mary Duff, knew about both recent hysterectomies. She visited the maternity unit to see the two patient files. She was not made welcome and the reaction to her questions was defensive. It was as if her presence was considered trespass. But this time Ciara brought her the two charts. They had been on Ciara's desk overnight, but oddly one of the histology reports was now missing. After getting a copy of the missing report from pathology, she reassured Ciara that something would be done.

Mary Duff then told the hospital's Medical Director, Mr Lennon. In turn he had just received a phone call from Donal O'Shea, the CEO of the Health Board, who had been briefed by the solicitor. The Health Board then moved with speed to establish if the perceptions of the two midwives deserved serious consideration. When the concerns were deemed valid, Dr Neary was invited to attend to discuss them. The following Tuesday, Dr Neary was asked to take administrative leave. Perhaps history was not going to repeat itself again in 1998.

Frighteningly, Judge Harding Clark tells us that Mary Duff did not know of the problem at the unit. Data provided to her the year before noted only one hysterectomy. This was a very isolated maternity unit. "Any concerns they kept to themselves, especially after the arrival of Mary Duff." But things were now changing; the knots were finally untangling. Or were they about to be tightened once again?

History Almost Repeats Itself

It was very difficult for management to remove Dr Neary from practice at the hospital. After Ann and Brigid's meeting with Gary Byrne, Dr Neary was asked to take two weeks' leave so that the allegations could be investigated. At the end of this period, Dr Neary wanted to return to work. But Dr Ambrose McLoughlin, the Assistant CEO of the Health Board, could not accept this. He wanted Dr Neary to be subject to a peer review of his caesarean hysterectomy rate between 1996 and 1998 and audited by the Institute of Obstetricians and Gynaecologists (IOG) of Ireland first.

Dr Neary agreed to this but later changed his mind. He argued, through his representatives, that peer review and audit while he was absent from the hospital would be so damaging to him that civil damages would not be sufficient remedy. Officials believed this was a threat to have them sacked. Dr Neary's advisors then obtained a copy of the files of the seventeen cases of caesarean hysterectomy they had identified during the period 1996–98. He had these cases reviewed by three established, eminent and practising consultant colleagues in Dublin. These doctors were approached on Dr Neary's behalf by Mr Finbarr Fitzpatrick of the Irish Hospital Consultants Association to provide reports.

The three obstetricians met with Dr Neary in one of their homes. They considered each of the files in turn. At all stages, they accepted the explanations provided by Dr Neary. Eight of the seventeen cases they were asked to review were excluded because Dr Neary said they were consent hysterectomies – necessitated because of the prohibition in the hospital of tubal ligations. He cited industrial relations difficulties as the reason why health board management wanted him out of the hospital. The doctors believed these explanations.

The three doctors produced two reports and concluded that "Dr Neary's practices were deemed to present no danger to patients" (*Lourdes Hospital Inquiry* Report p.6).

However, the health board was horrified by these reports. News spread rapidly in the hospital that Neary had been cleared by Dublin doctors. Because of the secrecy surrounding the reports, no one knew for sure what was going to happen. Neary returned to work in the unit with the now-panicked midwives who had revealed his practices.

But research of files and registers by the health board persuaded them that women were at high risk from Dr Neary's particular obstetric habits. He was now not permitted to perform a hysterectomy without obtaining a second opinion. So, in a very toxic environment, Dr Ambrose McLoughlin, supported by Mr Lennon and Mary Duff, on behalf of the health board, did something that had never happened before in this scandalous story's twenty-four-year history. They did the right thing, something that required a serious degree of moral courage. They followed through in the interests of women having babies. They supported "Ann" against an obstetrician.

They went abroad to seek the opinion of a British obstetrician, Dr Michael Maresh, a consultant in St Mary's Hospital, Manchester, on the same nine cases reviewed in Dublin. A significant number of consultants and other hospital personnel believed that Neary's suspension was contrived and formed part of a larger picture to rid the health board of consultants who held out for complete clinical independence. They received Dr Maresh's report on 7 December. Dr Maresh had a completely different view to the Dublin doctors.

Dr Maresh wrote:

From the information supplied I have major concerns about Dr Neary continuing to practise currently as a consultant obstetrician. His clinical judgement appears to be significantly impaired and women appear to be being put at risk. Although my concerns relate mainly to his excessive use of hysterectomy post delivery I do have concerns of other aspects of his management of patients. In addition to his clinical judgement I have concerns about his skills at caesarean section currently if there are complications. Finally, Dr Neary's perception of events appears impaired.

Tragically many of these women who were deprived of having children in future were young. Three were having their first baby. One of the three lost her baby (through no fault of Dr Neary) and so now will never have children of her own.

Having considered Dr Maresh's report, the CEO invoked appendix IV of the Consultants' Contract and instructed Dr Neary to take immediate administrative leave with effect from 11 December 1998. However, it was difficult to deliver this instruction to Dr Neary. The letterbox of his home was sealed. In the end they succeeded and the tightly tied knots supporting Neary were unwinding at last.

On 14 December, full details of the nine cases reviewed by Dr Maresh were published in *The Irish Times*. This is how most of the women learned for the first time of the hospital's and Neary's dark secret. The outside world knew at last.

The Medical Council became involved after the newspaper reported. They wrote to the NEHB requesting details. The health board forwarded documentation to them in January 1999 and the name of Michael Neary was temporarily removed from the Medical Register by the High Court on 5 February, with effect from 17 February. The Council decided that a *prima facie* case existed for the holding of a Fitness to Practise inquiry. This time, the mistakes of history were not repeated in the Lourdes Hospital.

All of the women, Niamh, Cathriona, Nicola, Noreen, Fidelma, Caitlin, to name but a few, wish to look out for "Ann". The woman who finally undid this abuse of power and trust is loved by them. Respect – earned, deserved and not sought – is their whispered thank you gift to her.

Part 1

One in a Million to One in Twenty

Nicola's Story

Nicola is sitting by her bed in Our Lady of Lourdes Hospital, Drogheda. It is 1986. Early summer sun streams in through the windows of the maternity ward. It is the sort of day when there is warmth in the sun for the first time after winter and you know Ireland is the most special place on earth.

Nicola was admitted for bed rest and observation four days earlier. Her usual doctor wanted to ensure that everything was okay, because her blood pressure was high. She is nineteen years old, expecting her first baby in a few weeks' time. She is ready to go home, reading a book to pass the time until a doctor tells her she can go. She is looking forward to her baby, not expecting it for a while because all first babies are late, everyone tells her.

In the meantime, her husband's twenty-first birthday is in a few days' time. They have things to do for that. They have great plans for the day. Nicola works in a florist's and loves it. A short distance away, their cottage nestles among the drumlin countryside of County Monaghan. Camellia trees, with their milky porcelain cup blossoms, are in full bloom in their garden. Her dad cares for it at the moment. If this early summer weather holds, they will have the celebrations under the trees.

For now, she roots in her bag to check that she still has the change to ring James. He is waiting for her call, expecting to collect her.

Her usual doctor is not available this morning. That is how she meets Dr Neary. He is simply the doctor on ward rounds that day.

She hears him before she can see him. A voice you listen to announces his arrival at the ward. Her bed is by the door. He stands tall at her bed, nurses and young doctors following. The grey-haired man lifted her chart from the neat bed's end, glanced at its details. He is clearly in charge, this man, and already he is placing his hand on her tummy.

"She's for a section straight away. Prepare her for theatre. I must do it today." He addresses the nurse. Then he turns to Nicola. "You have severe pre-eclampsia, toxaemia."

"Today! You want to do a section today?" This is Nicola's question to the man with the big hands who stands over her. She is alarmed now.

"It can't wait," he says, his tone brisk and in charge.

"Will my baby be okay?" Panic is welling up in her now.

"You're young; you'll have plenty more." He is gone as quickly as he arrived, and with him go the nurses and doctors.

Nicola is alone now. She wonders why, during the last few days in the hospital, no one gave her to understand that anything serious was wrong. Any time she asked, she was told she was "grand". She expected to go home. She wants to go home. She doesn't want to go to theatre and have her baby delivered before it is ready to be born.

She rings her husband at work. He is worried too, but they think the doctor must be right. Very reluctantly, they decide they have no choice but to accept the doctor's advice.

James arrives at the hospital and walks to the lift with Nicola as she is wheeled to theatre. By now it is about 2 p.m. Everyone in theatre is wearing green gowns. Nicola's name is on the board. They are waiting for her. Waiting to deliver her baby. She will always remember the counting down from 100, 99, 98, 97 . . . as the anaesthetic takes effect and as she falls asleep.

Next she knows, she is waking up in the ward. It is about four or five in the afternoon.

James is waiting for her. "We have a baby boy," he says. He doesn't tell her she had a hysterectomy. He wants to, but he can't. Nicola does not talk but reaches out and touches him. James knows that his young wife has lost her voice, and he does not know how to mouth the word "hysterectomy" either.

James is with her much of the time during these silent days. He wants to be sure he is there when Neary comes in and tells her; when Neary tells her that he, James, signed a consent form for the removal of her womb; that he was in the waiting room expecting news of their baby's birth when a nurse ran down the corridor to him, dressed in bluish green theatre garb, saying he had to come with her quickly. Dr Neary wanted to see him in the theatre immediately. James did as he was bid and followed this nurse.

Dr Neary came out of the theatre and spoke to him.

"Your wife had a massive bleed and has only an hour to live unless I remove her womb." Neary told James this terrible news at the theatre door. *"I need your consent to remove her womb or else she will be dead in an hour."*

James said okay as Dr Neary wiped his brow. James thought the blood on Neary's gloves and gown might be Nicola's. This frightened him; he thought only of his wife now and wanted Neary to get back into the theatre to do what was needed to save her. James was grateful to Neary as he watched him disappear through the theatre doors to save Nicola's life.

Later that evening, James met the doctor in the car park as they both left the hospital. *"She was one in a million,"* Neary told him. It was only the second time it had happened to him, he said.

"I nearly lost her," Neary repeated. *"Don't tell your wife. I'll do that."*

Three days later Dr Neary is on rounds again. James has just nipped out for a few minutes to get a 7-Up. Neary is at Nicola's bed again. She expects to be checked over.

He stands at her bed, nurses and young doctors in attendance on him.

"This is the lady who turned my hair grey," he says. They laugh at his little joke. *"You're an awful lucky woman to be sitting in this bed. This never happened to me except once before. You're one in a million,"* he says. *"You had a massive uncontrollable bleed, and placenta percretia. The placenta was growing outside your womb and when it was removed the wall of the womb crumbled with it. I had to do a hysterectomy."*

Nicola does not know what a hysterectomy is. But she

knows she has received two units of blood. She must look blank because Neary then says, "I had to remove your uterus."

Nicola cannot speak; she can hardly breathe. She reacts with silence. She can't say the word "hysterectomy".

For fourteen years after, she cannot say the word. Not to her husband, mother, beloved dad. It is as if her tongue was removed that day in 1986 and she has to learn to speak again. But she finds her voice again. When she does, we all applaud, quietly inside so no one else will know.

Of all the women in our group, Nicola was the youngest at the time of her hysterectomy. Neary was found guilty of professional misconduct in her case.

1

A Doctor is Named

In April 1996, I heard Dr Tony O'Sullivan on the very popular morning radio show hosted by Gay Byrne. Gay was then arguably Ireland's most popular radio and television personality. Tony, an Irish GP recently returned from Britain, was talking about the harm that can sometimes befall patients while in hospital and the difficulty they experience when they or their relatives seek an explanation. He wanted to develop a database of listeners' experiences of such injury. He asked people to contact him.

I was very interested in his request and wanted to help. I had a background in law and sociological research, so I thought this might be useful. I wrote to Tony and, with a small number of other volunteers, we set to work attempting to find out what patients' experiences were like. Forty people wrote to Tony in the weeks following his radio interview. We set about trying to help them. That is how I became involved in what Tony described as patient advocacy.

In the following two years we wrote annual reports detailing the sad experiences of the patients and their relatives who contacted us. This included complaints to the Medical Council from a small number of former patients alleging inappropriate sexual examinations by a consultant at Our Lady of Lourdes Hospital in Drogheda, Dr Michael Shine, when they were teenagers. Complaints had also been made to the Gardaí.

I was interviewed by Paul Maguire about the 1997 annual report in early October 1998. Paul was the presenter of *Loose Talk*, a morning current affairs show on LMFM, the local radio station for Louth and Meath. Two months later, just before Christmas 1998, I got another phone call from LMFM, asking if I would talk to Paul again about the lead story in *The Irish Times* that morning.

"Have you seen it?" asked the researcher. "It's about a doctor, an obstetrician who has been placed on administrative leave because he is accused of removing the wombs of young women just after they have a baby." Rumours had been circulating in the area in the week before so they suspected the story related to a doctor in their local hospital, Our Lady of Lourdes in Drogheda.

"No," I say, "I haven't seen it yet."

"Two midwives made a complaint about him. He hasn't been named, neither has the hospital, so we have to be very careful," she said. "They said he recently removed the womb of a twenty-year-old girl just eighteen minutes after she had her baby. An English professor who reviewed nine other women's cases said this was part of a pattern and his practice was not safe for women."

"That's dreadful," I said. "Do the women know?"

"They're being told at the moment," she said, "by their GPs. Will you talk to Paul about the effect this will have on young women hearing this news today, from your experience of supporting people who had bad experiences in hospital?"

"Okay, I'll try my best."

"Talk generally. Just like when you were on in October. I'll ring back in ten minutes," she said and replaced the phone.

I had a quick look at this terrifying lead story, written by Alison O'Connor and Mark Brennock. It seems that while the student midwives were expressing their concerns about this unnamed doctor in this unnamed hospital, back at the maternity unit he was removing the womb of another young woman who was thirty-three weeks pregnant. I had never heard of the procedure the paper was calling a "caesarean hysterectomy".

When the interview started Paul asked how young women who had hysterectomies after giving birth would feel this morning on hearing this news.

"For many it would be a dreadful shock. The last place you expect to be injured is in a hospital and by a doctor," I said. "Young patients have particular difficulties when medical injury occurs. Naturally they have had a huge need to put their life back together, especially a healthy young person. They have a job to do, they need to develop careers, go to college, form relationships, get married. Young mothers will have their baby to mind. This can stop them thinking through their experiences. In later life these problems could come back for resolution."

I spoke too about a lack of dignity, respect and informed consent as huge issues for damaged patients, how medical treatment was often felt as assault by patients and the difficulty the medical profession has in understanding these concepts.

As the interview was ending Paul asked, "Can I give your number to women if they ring, as I expect they will?"

"Of course," I said.

After this interview my phone started to ring. Over the course of the next few days, six women rang me to tell me about their terrible births and other stories. One name and one hospital kept recurring. Four had had caesarean hysterectomies in their teens or twenties. Two were older women in their forties or fifties who experienced damaging gynaecological surgery. Three had been contacted by their GPs and were the cases spoken of in *The Irish Times*. I will never forget these voices at the end of the phone: young voices, country voices, quiet voices, older ones too. All women. Some quietly angry, most flat as if drained of all energy, all shocked, grief-struck. I would come to recognise each voice very well indeed; come to know its owner with a rare depth. We would come to know each other with the intimacy of people who share a terrible secret. All were patients in the same hospital; all but one were patients of the same doctor.

I would get a chance to read *The Irish Times* reports in great detail over that week leading up to Christmas. I read about the midwives' concerns, the refusal by the doctor, supported by his representative from the Irish Hospital Consultants Association (IHCA), Finbarr Fitzpatrick, to accept the concerns when they were put to him by North Eastern Health Board officials. Furthermore, three colleagues who reviewed nine of his cases were not critical of him and a subsequent review by an English professor found serious concerns with the doctor's caesarean hysterectomy practice. This led to the health board writing to the doctor and asking him to take paid administrative leave pending a review of his practice by the Institute of Obstetricians and Gynaecologists of Ireland.

One young voice, Nicola's, is hard to forget. She rang because she heard "the unnamed doctor" and the "unnamed maternity unit" were to be identified on national TV on RTÉ's respected current affairs programme *Prime Time* that same evening. She apologised for disturbing me and then told me her sad and terrible story. A doctor had told her she would not be going home in a box because he saved her life. He told her she was one in a million; only once before had a young woman in his care lost her womb having a baby.

She hoped against hope that the doctor under suspension was not her doctor. Otherwise it might all have been unnecessary. She was not one of the women in *The Irish Times*, she said, or at least she did not think so.

"The town is agog that it was him," she said, still not naming him. I was worried about her because her husband, James, was at work at the time of her call.

After the screening of the *Prime Time* programme and the naming of the doctor, she rang back.

"It's him," she said, slow and shocked. "It's Dr Neary in Our Lady of Lourdes."

I tried to reassure her that this didn't mean her operation was unnecessary. "Maybe you needed it, Nicola; you probably did. Probably most of the operations he did were necessary. Your case is not in the paper." I didn't know who I was persuading, myself or Nicola. She needed her hope. I hope I left it with her that evening.

"Wait till James hears," she said. Her child needed her attention. She had to go to him.

I did not know where this story would finally lead, or that Tony and I would hear variations of this story over and over. I would never get used to it. Each story different, each one the same. Each new voice sending my heart into my toes as together we tried to make sense of the chaos.

It was a terrible Christmas for the six women who phoned me at this time when grief and shock are always deeper, always isolating. I know because they told me. It would be the first of many difficult Christmases.

Cathriona's Story

Cathriona is the tender warrior of the group. She became Neary's worst nightmare. She is from Kells, a modern Irish town with a rich royal and ecclesiastical history. Perhaps that is why this young woman instinctively understands the value of justice and the healing properties of truth-telling and bearing witness. She knows how to harness their immense power to heal herself and the other women in the group. She understands the importance of the group, too. Her instinct is to roll up her sleeves and help anyone in pain, and that's what she did then. Cathriona is married to Danny. Neary removed her womb and one ovary when she was twenty-five years old.

She was one of the first women to consult a solicitor. In fact, she did this before the news ever broke about Michael Neary. Her natural instinct surfaced to protect her and her new baby. At first she had little luck and met the usual obstacles. The first solicitor she consulted discouraged her, telling her that if she lost her case she would lose her house, and furthermore he would charge her £100 an hour for this advice. He wanted her to sign documents to this effect. Cathriona was a twenty-five-year-old woman who had just bought her first home. She and her husband were busy doing up their lovely cottage, putting together a home for their two children. To right a grievous wrong, she would have to sign this all away before it began. She couldn't even get her records from the hospital four months before the story broke. She then changed solicitor just before the news broke.

In fact, Cathriona never wanted to be Neary's patient for her second baby. She attended him when pregnant with her first child Justin, but for some reason didn't like him. But when she went into the Lourdes in the early morning of 31 January 1996, she was in labour. Her baby was not coming as quickly as expected, so they put her on a drip to help things along. All day she worked until she was exhausted. At about 11 p.m. it was decided she needed an emergency section. She has told what happened to her many times so that the world will know, take heed and take steps to prevent another Drogheda.

"Before I knew it, I was in a gown and going to theatre on a trolley. The nurse told me to say goodbye to my husband. I said why? Am I going to die? My epidural was topped up and my baby was born by section at ten to twelve. Almost midnight. I heard a call for Dr Neary at about midnight. I didn't know it was for me."

Cathriona wasn't aware anything bad was happening. She asked about her baby and was told all was well. They then said she was bleeding. Then, as she told the Medical Council, "I was aware of nothing 'til I woke about one o'clock." She looked at the clock. "A doctor spoke to me. 'Do you know we removed your womb?' I said no."

This was Dr Neary. He spoke to her parents and her husband, who had been with her all that long day. Cathriona was in recovery and getting some blood.

"I did not meet Dr Neary for a good few days. I ran into him in the corridor. 'We keep missing each other,' he said. He told me I had had a very traumatic experience. It was a nightmare and I should go home and forget it."

That was all he said to Cathriona but he had spoken to her husband and parents. She understood from them that it had been a life-saving operation. Neary had to do it to save her life. It was so urgent, he never asked consent from her young husband.

After she went home, Cathriona was delighted with baby Seamus, but she avoided her friends. "I felt it was my fault I'd had a hysterectomy at twenty-five. I didn't want anyone to know I'd had it. I felt like a freak but I got on with my life. I felt lucky to have my two children but I could never get away from it."

Eight weeks after her baby was born, Cathriona went to Neary for her post-natal check up. He told her she was a nightmare case, lucky to be alive. She tried to talk to him and ask him what had happened.

"Well, it wasn't cancer anyway," *he said, diverting her questions. He added,* "At least I have sorted your family planning problems." *After this Cathriona was totally shocked and left the room.*

"I couldn't believe a man like that would say that to me, at twenty-five years of age, not to have any more kids, and that was the sympathy I got."

Cathriona asked her GP, not Neary, why she had had the hysterectomy. Her GP had a letter from Neary saying he had spent the whole night in theatre with her. She didn't remember him there at all.

Cathriona then went to another solicitor, who tried to get her medical notes. Shortly after, in December 1998, Cathriona was phoned by her GP. He said he had been contacted by the health board. Her case was in The Irish Times. *Seemingly her pathology notes did not back up what Neary said. In her files, Neary had written that there was a rupture in her womb. There was none according to her pathology record.*

Cathriona felt totally robbed. She would have loved more babies. Despite her robust personality and great family, she found it very hard. The Medical Council found Neary guilty of professional misconduct in her case.

2

Quiet and Clamour

The first meeting with the six women was in a secluded place. We chose a country house hotel, the Boyne Valley, at the end of a tree-lined avenue, just outside Drogheda. No unwelcome guests were likely, no prying eyes.

Dr Tony O'Sullivan and I drove to Drogheda that winter's evening, very unsure of what lay ahead. Our plan was to ensure people were safe. We asked them not to come alone. We would tell them of the services the health board had put in place for them, but mostly we would just introduce ourselves. It was a chance to have a look at each other.

A few days earlier, I had phoned the North Eastern Health Board (NEHB) to find out how they planned to assist the women through this trauma. Tony and I felt it was important that services were put in place for them and it would be helpful if I could tell them some good news at the meeting.

First I got on to the communications office. That was a total waste of time. I got some PR spiel. This really annoyed me so I rang the CEO's office direct. I left a message with his secretary. I said women had been phoning me and wanted to know what the board was doing to help them. Before I got back into my kitchen, the phone rang. It was Ambrose McLoughlin, Deputy CEO of the NEHB. I couldn't believe it. He said he wanted to help, that services were being put in place for the women, including a second independent medical opinion, counselling, any extra medical care. They had already set up the helpline and many women had called it.

"The health board has a duty to do this, to look after the women," he said. He wanted to work with Tony and me. He expressed sympathy for the women. He was glad they were meeting each other. He offered to meet any of them who wanted to meet him. He was prioritising the early sending out of their records so that they could consult another doctor for an opinion. "Tell them that from me at the meeting," he added.

This was great news. The health board was very helpful, and at such a senior level.

We arrived at the Boyne Valley early and ordered coffee in the dimly lit lounge. A young couple dressed in outdoor winter clothes looked in but decided against coming in. So did another.

"Do you think that's them?" I asked Tony.

"I don't know. They look very young," he said.

They were.

We had booked the Georgian room. Chairs were neatly laid out in rows in this elegant high-ceilinged room with its velvet drapes. A table with a crisp white table cloth was laid with cups and saucers for the tea and coffee we ordered. Ten people were waiting for us inside. Every woman was supported by a man.

"Let's rearrange the seats," said Tony. "We can introduce ourselves better that way." In no time we were sitting in a semicircle. Then another couple joined us and stayed slightly to the back. Everyone was here.

Tony introduced himself and me. "You introduce yourselves when you're ready and only then," Tony said. "I'm a GP with an interest in women's health and in helping damaged patients."

Damaged patients: a strange concept that did not seem out of place here. But everyone did introduce themselves to us. They decided to trust two people they had never met before, to whom they had only spoken on the phone. For some reason they must have liked the look of us.

Even as Cathriona, May, Noreen, Clodagh, Nicola and Sara and their husbands told us their names, there was a sense of shocked and broken hearts in this room, of lives torn apart. Three of the women had been pregnant with their first babies, one with her second, when Neary took out their wombs. One very quiet young woman also had both ovaries removed by Dr Neary. He had been a danger to three women in the room at least. They were women whose care had been seriously criticised in the Maresh Report. Neary had removed their wombs unnecessarily, the report said. Two of the women were older. Their lives, they said, had been seriously damaged by the gynaecological care they received in Our Lady of Lourdes.

There was a shyness in the room. But still Sara, one of the young women, spoke. "I read my story in the paper. The details of what happened to me and my baby were printed for all to see and I knew nothing about it. What about patient confidentiality?"

"You can't trust any of them," her husband beside her said.

Nicola spoke up. "My GP phoned me and asked me to visit him. When I got down to see him, he told me there were queries about Dr Neary doing too many hysterectomies. I could not believe it. I trusted Dr Neary. But then my GP said he always had worries about what had happened to me but was afraid to say because I was very upset when my baby was born. He told me to get *The Irish Times*."

"The health board leaked the files," another said. "Do you know how the paper got them?"

"We have no idea who told the press. But the health board say they didn't do it."

I told them of my first experiences with the health board and of Ambrose McLoughlin's offer of help.

"We got it in writing yesterday," Tony said. "Written promises."

That evening Tony and I listened to the stories of the six women and their husbands who sat before us on a cold dark January night in a hotel that was practically empty except for us. It was mostly the women who spoke. The men, silent in their support, asked very few questions. They really just wanted to listen and then to talk, some a little, others much more, as the night wore on.

"I loved being pregnant," one of the young women told us all, "and now that's all over and maybe no need for it all."

"People in the area are supporting him," one of the men said. "Saying he was a great doctor, he could do no wrong, it must all be a mistake."

"You can expect that," Tony said, "but pay no attention. You will find that as time goes by some of the women loudest in his support may even join us. They will come to their senses. Some of them are in denial."

Tony answered medical questions explaining the procedure, how blood loss was estimated during a birth, etc.

"You will need your medical records to find out about your own operation," he said.

"I can't get mine out of them," Nicola said. "Every time I phone the hospital I am told my notes are in the post but they don't turn up. They're just trying to get me off the phone."

"I tried to get my records from the hospital last August because I was very upset about the way my labour was managed," Cathriona told us. "My child was in distress during my labour too. But I couldn't get them until now. They never even answered my solicitor until this week. Time is running out for me to take a case. I have to start things very soon but I'm afraid I could lose my house. Last year another solicitor asked me to sign my house away. And he wanted a hundred pounds an hour for his advice. How can ordinary people afford this? When this news broke I got a new solicitor. He's different."

"I can help you with getting your records if you want," I said. "After you write in and ask for them I can follow up on your behalf, do the harassing, make sure they find them for you. I can find out who is the right person to contact too."

"You have a legal right to your records now," Tony added. "Under the Freedom of Information Acts. In health board hospitals, they have to give you your files." They did not know that. "I will ask some colleagues to help if that is what you want – obstetricians to give you their opinion on your surgery. Then you will know if your operations were needed. They will send the bill to the health board, so no money will need to change hands." They wanted this.

Women then started to speak a little about what happened to them during the birth of their first or second baby, about the circumstances surrounding the removal of their wombs and ovaries. Many of the stories were the same.

"At my six-week check up Dr Neary told me he solved my family planning problems," Cathriona told us. "I was twenty-five years of age. He said I was a nightmare case. He frightened my husband and family to death."

"I never even got a blood transfusion and he told me I was in danger of bleeding to death. I was awake because I had an epidural and I asked him was he sure. There was nothing I could do." Sara told us.

"He just kept poking at me during my operation," one woman said.

Clodagh, the quiet young woman at the back, said very quietly, "Three women had caesarean sections the week I had my womb removed and all three had hysterectomies too."

"That's extraordinary," Tony said. "Very extraordinary. Caesarean hysterectomy is very rare, a life-saving operation. Three in the one week in a small enough hospital. This must be a matter for the Medical Council."

Tony explained to the women that the Medical Council is the body that deals with complaints against doctors. He suggested they may need to write to them. They did not know this either, that there was somewhere to complain about a doctor.

At night's end, we sipped on the by-now cold tea. We had no appetite for the biscuits. The women and their husbands chatted quietly to each other. Some exchanged phone numbers and two talked of their surprise at seeing each other there. They were neighbours. Faces were put on the names and voices for me that winter night.

"It's strange to hear other women telling my story. I thought it was only me, that I was one in a million, a nightmare case, but it happened to someone else I know in January 1996," Cathriona told us.

Tony and I were quiet in the car on the way home. Images of women damaged in a profound way floated through my mind. I thought about a string of pearls ripping and each single pearl falling one by one to the floor. Their backs were breaking, like that string of pearls, by the force of the news.

Cathriona rang a few days later to say she had taken her notes to her GP. He told her there were discrepancies between the pathology findings and Neary's report of events. "The pathologist said there was no rupture of my womb. I am issuing legal proceedings."

Another followed a few days later with a similar story and was to consult the same solicitor. It was important to move quickly, as the time was running out, she said. "Papers need to be lodged in the High Court to stop the clock ticking." This was a reference to the Statute of Limitations – a three-year time limit which then existed on taking legal action in cases of medical negligence.

While some women grieved quietly and in private for what Neary did to them and their families, others marched loudly and publicly in support of their hero doctor.

Cathriona wrote in early February:

Sorry for not being in contact since the meeting. I have been having a bad time for the last few weeks. I am continually getting mouth ulcers and feeling dead tired. Everything is being played over and over like a tape in my head. I am trying to put things to the background until it crops up again. I still have to be examined by a doctor to confirm what I have and what I do not have.

She enclosed a copy of a *Drogheda Independent* report into a march held in support of Dr Neary a few weeks earlier. "There is another march being organised again this week for Dr Neary, this time to Leinster House. A bus has been organised for anyone who wants to go." She signed off saying, "I am sorry I sound all doom and gloom."

I had heard of these marches but nothing prepared me for the tone of Marie Kierans' article. Neary is not named, though his name was widely known by then.

In the rain and cold they came in their hundreds last Thursday night. Women of all ages, some on their own and many accompanied by husbands and children, gathered in Fair Street to participate in the protest walk over what they see as the unfair treatment of the consultant obstetrician at the centre of the caesarean hysterectomy investigation.

A thousand people left the warmth and comfort of their homes to express their solidarity for the doctor.

They came from both sides of the river Boyne and from the small villages scattered throughout mid-Louth and East Meath, a mixture of age groups and backgrounds, but all with a common bond – to show their support for the doctor and express their anger at his treatment at the hands of the Lourdes hospital and North Eastern Health Board, and their concern over the leakage of his name and patient medical records to the media.

The turnout, bigger than the support group had anticipated, made its way in a calm and dignified manner over Fair Street, onto the North Road, then to the side entrance of the hospital where a letter and list of questions was handed in to a representative of the North Eastern Health Board by a delegation of four supporters. . . . The support group initially started with eighteen patients but numbers have escalated in recent weeks culminating in the walk last Thursday night.

The huge numbers showed *"the level of concern that exists locally over the situation and also reflects the high level of esteem in which the doctor is held by his patients,"* one marcher said, and another is quoted as saying:

"The turnout here tonight has endorsed our decision to set up a support group. People might say that there is apathy out there but the people of Drogheda have proved that when they believe in something they are prepared to stand up and be counted. We are not going to stop now until we have answers and further action is being planned."

The article then stated as fact that *"The number of cases under investigation is now down to six."* The article also quoted a statement by the NEHB defending itself against accusations that it leaked patient files to the media:

"The Board cannot remain silent when it is suggested that patient records at one of its hospitals are not secure. Patients need to know that their records are absolutely secure – and that the Board has neither released, leaked or authorised the release or leak of any confidential data."

The article ended in the same vein as it began:

Meanwhile, although the doctor at the centre of the investigation did not take part in the walk, it is understood that he visited a well known hostelry at the outskirts of town afterwards where he received a standing ovation from the packed pub.

"That was the Monasterboice Inn, his local," Cathriona said later. "That's what they are saying round here anyway. He has his lunch there every day. Can you believe it?"

Marie Kierans and Niall Moonan wrote a further article giving an indication of how Dr Neary was feeling about this. A "close friend" was speaking about him.

The Drogheda Independent *has learned that the doctor at the centre of the Inquiry* [the Institute of Obstetricians and Gynaecologists Inquiry set up after revelations were made about Neary's caesarean hysterectomy rate] *is determined to clear his name after being deeply moved by a support march for him in Drogheda last Thursday. The consultant according to a close friend was "overwhelmed" by the 1,000-strong crowd which turned out for the walk in protest at the way in which he has been treated by the North Eastern Health Board and the Lourdes Hospital.*

The article continued: *"The doctor's morale was greatly boosted by the march turnout according to a close friend."* The article went on to quote the close friend:

"Obviously it has been a very difficult couple of months for the doctor. He has had to watch his name being blackened in the media, and at times his morale was very low. But the response from ordinary members of the public in recent weeks encouraged him greatly and has made him even more determined to clear his name. He said to me the other day that it is only when you are in trouble you realise who your friends are, and thankfully he has many. He is particularly delighted that all the good work he has done down through the years has not been forgotten. . . . He fully stands by the caesarean hysterectomies that he carried out," said the close friend.

Doubts were thrown on the inquiry and its ability to do its work because of legal difficulties, mentioned earlier in *Irish Medical News*, the Drogheda paper said. The medical news article is quoted as claiming that *"the IOG and the group due to conduct the clinical review is concerned that the inquiry would not have legal privilege, and as a result members of the inquiry team could leave themselves open to being sued.*" These concerns were dispelled by the NEHB, however, the article stated. The board denied also and condemned suggestions that patient files had been leaked by them to the media. Details of a further march to the Department of Health the following week and a contact number for the doctor's support group was included at the end of the article.

The paper also published photographs of the crowd holding banners with slogans such as:

"We want Dr Neary back"
(his name was blacked out here, of course)

"Patients outraged files released to the media"

A sweet little boy of three or four years wearing a gorgeous check cap was photographed holding a placard reading, *"We want Dr Neary back"*.

Is it any wonder Cathriona was depressed and upset? This was what appeared in local papers at the same time as victims of this doctor wrote their very painful letters of complaint to the Medical Council in January 1999. Three of the women sent their complaints about Neary to me to forward to the Medical Council. I placed all three letters in one large brown envelope for delivery at the end of January. The process of finding out the truth had begun. Perhaps too, the process of rethreading that string of pearls with even stronger thread.

Tony and I received letters too – in support of Neary. Thirty or so. Most, but not all, were signed and addressed. One described a first-time mother's continuing trust in Neary, despite the revelations. *"During my dealings with Dr Neary I have found him to be reassuring, understanding and caring. In fact my only reason for attending the Lourdes Hospital for my son's birth was that Dr Neary practised there . . . if I am fortunate enough to have another baby I will certainly attend Dr Neary."* Neary attended this birth the day after he performed his last caesarean hysterectomy and the day the midwives raised their concerns with the legal advisor to the NEHB.

Another woman sent us a copy of a handwritten letter she wrote to the NEHB about Dr Neary: *"in 1997 I asked him outright to perform a hysterectomy but he refused saying that he didn't believe in unnecessary surgical procedures . . . In the light of the above I found it very difficult to believe the allegations that are being made against him."*

A third letter is to Dr Tony O'Sullivan: *"I wish to express my support for Dr Neary in the strongest possible way . . . Had Dr Neary not acted with the speed that was required, I might not be round to see this sad indictment of a wonderful man . . . Like thousands of other women I want my doctor back."*

Despite this support, however, the Medical Council acted. We thought they must have received our complaints. They suspended Neary from the medical register pending a Fitness to Practise Inquiry in early February 1999. This meant he could not legally practice, in a private capacity, while on leave. We knew he was practising. He was referring patients for blood tests and for admission to the Lourdes. He was stopped by his peers.

I phoned the hospital over and over about Nicola's files. She herself had been trying since before Christmas. By late

February they had not turned up, despite several reassurances that they were in the post. This difficulty was poisoning my attitude to the Health Board.

"I know how to make a pest of myself. I'm prepared to sit in the foyer of Our Lady of Lourdes hospital if necessary to get these notes," I said to Jim Reilly, the official I had most contact with. Jim was the main point of contact with the women. He was charged with providing them with the services they needed, such as a second opinion, counselling, etc.

"We don't want you to have to do that," he said.

Instead of this direct action we decided to take the Deputy CEO Ambrose McLoughlin and Jim Reilly up on their offer of a meeting. Nicola was up for it. We travelled to Kells for an 11 a.m. meeting in early March, a very pleasant spring day. I was very, very nervous indeed. I brought my husband, Wilfie Blackwood, as driver because I did not feel up to driving myself. We arrived at the offices in Kells in good time and Nicola and her husband James were there before us. Looking back now, I know this was a test of Ambrose and Jim for Nicola and James. They needed to walk the walk now. Find Nicola's notes or they were dead.

We sat in the reception of the insignificant single-storey building, waiting for the officials. We laughed out of nerves as time passed. This is Nicola's way, as I had come to know. Staff came and went, obviously having their coffee break. After about half an hour a tall, slender man came out.

"I'm Jim Reilly," he said in a gentlemanly way. "You're welcome to Kells. We're really sorry for the delay but we hope to be with you very soon."

We were watching our manners so we just nodded as we all shook hands. Sometime later he appeared again and asked us to join him and Ambrose in a nearby room. We followed him in to the bland meeting room and took our places on one side of the table from the two officials. Ambrose McLoughlin stood as we entered and extended a strong hand in greeting, the kind of handshake where the body comes too.

Ambrose took charge of the meeting from the off. "We have the hospital records for you at last," he said, handing them to Nicola and addressing us all after introductions were completed and tea and coffee poured. "We were waiting for them to arrive."

I got the impression that they were not sure they would be available until the very last minute. There was tension and anxiety in the room and it wasn't all coming from us.

James asked, "Why do you think Neary did what he did to young women? It's as if he hijacked Nicola. She was sitting at the bed expecting to come home when he said she needed to go to the theatre. How many women and families did he do this to?" He looked at his wife sitting beside him. She nodded in agreement.

There was no answer from Ambrose to James's "why" but this didn't seem like an evasion of the question because of the animated engagement of this big man with James and Nicola. "We know of sixty-seven cases and it could be as many as 165. The initial review was conducted on nine cases but these were selected by Neary himself. They were not complete files, and only Neary's descriptions of the procedures were taken into account." This was a reference to the three Irish obstetricians who had said there were no problems with Neary.

"Who are they anyway and what were they doing supporting him?" James asked Ambrose.

"That's an official secret. The reports of these good men are locked away in a safe. No one has seen them but our CEO and legal advisor. Finbarr Fitzpatrick of the IHCA refused to accept that Neary was a risk to patients and asked these three eminent doctors to do it. It caused awful trouble for the midwives who told us what Neary was up to. We couldn't get him out of the hospital after that. We couldn't stop him operating on women.

"I am only interested in three things," he went on. "Patients, patients, patients. But the culture in the hospital was doctor-driven. This must change. It's patients who matter. We will go back as far as needed to find out the truth about this. Standards must improve; nurses are too subservient and patients too trusting. Women were not safe in this hospital. The doctor is sick. He still accepts no responsibility for the damage he caused. You just can't remove young women's wombs for no reason, full stop. The Review by the IOG is only a preliminary investigation. The real investigation will be by the statutory body." It took me a while to realise that he was talking about the Medical Council. "The facts of this case are so bad that one member of the board got sick at the meeting when the details were discussed. In the US, Neary would be charged with crimes."

I found it easy to agree with all this. I was glad this man was on our side and not against us. I was very glad he was so passionately engaged. Afterwards I realised that James and Nicola were equally impressed. They gave us about two and a half hours. There was a strong feeling that these officials had had a hard time and wanted to help. Jim Reilly, the quiet-spoken man at Ambrose McLoughlin's side, said, "The Medical Council has received your letters of complaint."

"That's where the important decisions will be made," Ambrose repeated with a confident nod of his head.

"Neary's supporters are silent now," he added as we stood to leave. He was referring to the marches outside the NEHB offices over Neary's removal. I thought of the letters we received from former patients of Neary saying how he saved their lives; and others from children saying how Neary was a wonderful man, that they would not be here without him and that his were the first hands that ever touched them.

But Nicola got her notes. The object of the exercise had been achieved. She and James could now find out about her operation.

Nicola rang some days later.

"I took my notes to the GP. She said she could see no reason why I needed a hysterectomy." My heart sank. Nicola spoke quickly, but her tone was matter-of-fact, revealing yet concealing her distress; telling the truth but trying to hide her pain.

I asked her how she was.

"Not a bother, how are you? James is upset though. He tried to get my notes after our baby was born. The door was closed in his face by a nurse in the hospital records office. They didn't care. He thinks they just thought he was dirt. The only one they cared about was the doctor." Before our conversation ended, she told me, "My pathology notes are missing. They are not in with the rest."

A little later James rang. A man of few but always very important words.

"Sheila, I'm very worried about Nicola. She never spoke about what happened to her that day. Do you think you could meet and speak to her in greater depth about it? I think she would talk to you."

"It would be a privilege," I said. "Get her to ring me."

There was a pause. "Why did he do it?" he asked, as he often did.

"I don't know, James. It is hard to understand it."

"Do you think he hated women?" he asked. "Do you think it was us, something about us? Do you think he thought we were fools and he could do what he wanted?"

"I don't know, James. Why do you think he did it?"

"I think he just wanted to and he could. He was king. What he said went. And those nuns and nurses were all over him, that's what I think."

Niamh's Story

Niamh was the youngest in our group, just turned twenty when she went into Our Lady of Lourdes Hospital to deliver her first baby in late 1998. A quiet-spoken girl, she is gentle and restrained in manner and word. It is impossible for me to imagine Niamh's voice raised in anger. It is impossible to imagine her hurting anyone. But she was brave. Days after she went home, she walked into Neary's private clinic to collect her file. She was very wise to do this, as we discovered later that many files could not be found.

From the first time I met her, she reminded me of my own slightly built, quiet-spoken nineteen-year-old daughter at home. Niamh, a girl with cowslip-coloured hair. She was much minded and loved by her mother, her partner and the other women in the group.

She was living in Scotland when she became pregnant but she decided to come back to Ireland when she was thirty-three weeks pregnant so she could have her baby close to home. She went to Dr Neary in his private clinic in Fair Street. Her mother made the appointment with Dr Neary for Niamh. Dr Neary had delivered Niamh herself twenty years before, so they had great trust and confidence in him. He had a history with them.

"I had been hearing his name all my life," Niamh said, "hearing how good he was." Niamh was telling her story to the Fitness to Practise Committee of the Medical Council. "He agreed to see me straight away because I was thirty-three weeks pregnant and my baby was in breach position. At my first appointment with him he told me the baby's head was not engaged and it mightn't happen now. I told him I was worried about this. The bypass around Drogheda was being built as well, so the roads were closed. I was afraid I might not be able get to the hospital. Dr Neary suggested admitting me for caesarean section and this suited me very well."

Niamh was admitted to the hospital the night before she was due to have her section. She asked for an epidural rather than a general anaesthetic. When she reached the theatre, a number of nurses and an anaesthetist were already there. Sean, her partner, was with her. Dr Neary helped Niamh onto the table for her surgery. He helped place her leg in position as the epidural was administered. He delivered her baby ten or fifteen minutes later.

"My baby was handed to the nurse to be washed immediately she was born at 12.47 p.m. I was delighted." Everything was quiet and relaxed. There was no sense of anxiety or drama. "I was lying waiting to be stitched up," Niamh explained, "and the nurse came back and said my baby was okay, just so as I would know she was healthy."

Then Dr Neary told her *"he would have to take out my womb. I asked what he was talking about. He said he could not stop the bleeding and he would have to take it out. If he didn't take it out I would be dead quite soon. I wasn't aware of anything untoward happening. I wasn't weak or anything. I felt better than I should have after having a baby. I was expecting the next conversation to be that I was finished and getting ready to go out. By now it was about ten minutes after my baby was born. Sean left the theatre to dress the baby and they wouldn't let him back in when all this was happening. I wasn't expecting a hysterectomy.*

"Dr Neary didn't ask for help from anyone before saying he had to remove my womb. He just asked for the hysterectomy kit and went ahead and did it there and then. I felt helpless as he did it. No one spoke up for me. I just asked him to do a bikini line cut and he did that for me. I was back in recovery at 1.30.

"I didn't get any blood," Niamh added. *"He just said he had to do it. I got two bags of blood later, I think, not at the time. Afterwards I didn't see Dr Neary. I was very upset but glad to be alive and that my baby was okay. I believed he saved my life. I did not get the opportunity in the hospital. He would come in on a quick visit. It was never the right time to sit down and talk about it."*

The only chance Niamh got to talk to Dr Neary about what happened was at her six-week check up. *"I decided I would wait 'til then,"* Niamh said.

The six-week check up was in his clinic in Fair Street. He said that *"there was a weakness in part of my womb, that it was spongy and that it came away with the placenta and caused the bleeding."* Dr Neary drew a diagram of what *happened for Niamh. "He said it was a miracle I carried the baby for so long because of the way [my womb] was. He said it might be to do with the cyst I had as a child. He left me feeling I was lucky my baby didn't die. He didn't fully explain what had happened.*

"I made an appointment for a smear but when I went back he was gone." His secretary told Niamh there was a conspiracy to get Neary out of the hospital.

None of the nurses at the hospital would talk to her about what had happened. She worried it might be cancer; no one reassured her. She thinks about it all the time. It was all right when she thought it was to save her life, but not when she found out that it wasn't necessary.

A midwife who was in theatre at the time of Niamh's delivery was very upset by what had happened. Sometime later the pathology report confirmed the midwife's anxieties. There was no abnormality in Niamh's womb. Neary was found guilty of professional misconduct in her case.

3

"The Whitewash Report"

During the months of February, March and April 1999, the women continued to meet in the Boyne Valley Hotel. Friendships were formed. They rang each other to provide support in what was a very hostile and disbelieving environment locally. Our meetings lasted late into the night, talking, asking questions of Tony, hearing details of Irish doctors who would help them by reviewing their records. The doctors who first agreed were Dr Peter Lenehan and Dr Mary Wingfield. A number refused to help, however. Others agreed initially but later changed their minds.

Slowly, one by one, more women were contacting us. Word was spreading. By Easter there were eighteen women in the group. Women met at school gates, at playgroups, at supermarkets, at swimming pools and football pitches. They quietly and carefully spread the word of the group in this way. The hospital gave out my telephone number, as did the LMFM radio station. We were in contact with the hospital at this stage about the search for records, with varying degrees of success. Some women received their records very quickly; others were not so lucky. We were careful to leave the initial approaches to the women themselves.

The group was growing slowly but surely in numbers and in trust of one another. Women were phoning the hospital seeking files and consulting GPs too. Reality was dawning too that a terrible scandal involving them and their families was unfolding, a scandal that would grow to cover the whole north-east of this country.

For one thing, it was becoming clear that Dr Neary had performed caesarean hysterectomies as far back as 1979. It was also clear that Dr Neary gave women one of three reasons for the caesarean hysterectomy: they had lost a massive amount of blood; they had a defect of the womb caused by a drug used by their own mother when she gave birth to them to dry up her milk; or the placenta was adhered to the womb, making it necessary to remove the womb.

Tony was very disturbed by these explanations. He felt these complications were very unlikely to occur in such high numbers in a relatively small hospital. He looked through the women's files at our late-night meetings and was dismayed with what he found. We were also becoming worried that some women could not get their files. They appeared to be missing. This was causing dreadful grief. People had no way of finding out whether or not their operation was needed.

We were awaiting the report of the review of Neary's practice established at the time of his removal from the hospital by the Institute of Obstetricians and Gynaecologists of Ireland. They also met in the Boyne Valley to consider Neary's treatment of the women who had caesarean hysterectomies between 1992 and 1998. We wrote to them to ask them to include the case of a young girl who had a caesarean hysterectomy at nineteen years in 1986. Our request was refused, as it was outside the terms of reference. The women wanted to contribute to the review by providing the team with their side of the story. This never happened and no reason was given for this decision.

Their report was presented to the board of the NEHB on Monday 26 April 1999. It was reported in *The Irish Times* the Saturday before. The key finding was:

> *In 18 (46.2%) of patients Dr Neary's decision to perform a peripartum, caesarean hysterectomy was not acceptable clinical practice. In 16 (41%) cases his practice was considered acceptable, and in the remaining five (12.8%) doubtful.*

The report contained other devastating figures:

> *On the data available to the Review Group, Dr Neary performed 708 caesarean sections from 1992 to 1998 inclusive and 39 peripartum caesarean hysterectomies. This gives a peripartum caesarean hysterectomy rate of 5%, i.e. one for every 20 caesarean sections . . . This is twenty times the rate recorded in one Dublin maternity hospital (National Maternity Hospital, Holles Street) . . . giving an incidence of one in 441 caesarean sections.*
>
> (Review Group Report, p. 6)

The report also concluded that in relation to Michael Neary's clinical practice:

- *There was a high incidence of caesarean section.*

- *There was a high incidence of peripartum caesarean hysterectomy.*

- *In several patients there was an overestimation of the amount of blood loss.*

- *The diagnosis of a morbidly adherent placenta or uterine abnormality may have been incorrect in a number of cases.*

- *Consultation with another colleague concerning the need for a caesarean hysterectomy rarely occurred.*

- *Dr Neary considered that his job would be in jeopardy if he had carried out tubal ligation rather than a hysterectomy for the purposes of sterilisation.*

- *Operation notes often described heroic measures unjustified by patient records.*

(Review Group Report, p. 26)

The CEO of the NEHB, Mr Donal O'Shea, made several comments on the findings of this report at the meeting of the Board on 26 April.

The first of these was the suggestion by Neary and the review group that some of these operations happened because there wasn't a sufficient blood supply in the hospital. "The fact is that at no time, on no single occasion, has there been a shortage of blood. It didn't happen."

The CEO also disputed the suggestion that one-third of these hysterectomies were in fact sterilisations. Dr Neary himself had confirmed to Health Board management on 27 October 1998 that he had not undertaken caesarean hysterectomy for the purpose of sterilisation and the patient notes make it clear this was never an issue in these cases. The code of ethics of Our Lady of Lourdes Hospital, Drogheda, he pointed out, was not unusual and paralleled the code in other voluntary hospitals which did not have the high frequency of caesarean hysterectomy.

The CEO announced to the board that, as a precautionary measure, the board was carrying out a systematic look back at all of Dr Neary's records prior to 1992. The CEO further stated that Dr Neary was on paid administrative leave and he was taking advice in this regard.

More women phoned with worries once the IOG Review Group Report became public. Each woman's story was as upsetting as the next. Young women whose wombs were removed as far back as 1976 were getting in touch, each nervous and reticent. I couldn't believe what I was hearing.

"I am sorry to be bothering you about this but I was a patient of Dr Neary's. I am sure there is no cause to be worried but I'm afraid that maybe I didn't need my womb removed," were typical opening words.

Once again it was first and second babies, women in their twenties or early thirties. They too were told that they were bleeding to death; they were a one-in-a-million case; he was in theatre all night. I never got used to this story. Over and over my heart would sink to my feet as the self-same expressions, reasons and excuses were mentioned.

One woman who called also spoke of a friend. "I'm not the worst. I know a woman that it happened to when she was a teenager, but she won't ring. She is afraid to find out."

"She probably will in her own time," I said, horrified at the thought of a second teenage patient.

Grief and fear in the whole community was growing. My role was to listen but reassure. "Your operation could have been needed," I'd always say to the callers with their still-young voices at the end of the phone.

It was at this time too that I heard of women who were not told of their hysterectomy until their post-natal check up.

"He told me when my baby was ten weeks old, at my check up," Majella told me. I couldn't believe my ears. She'd had a caesarean but never knew of the hysterectomy. She was a private patient in a public ward in 1980. Neary visited her several times but never told her. "My husband was outside in the car waiting for me," she said. "I went out screaming to him. I wanted to get Neary then, but no one would listen to me. I went to a solicitor but I got nowhere."

Later on, Majella would say, "I could have stopped the whole thing if only I'd been braver." Of course she couldn't, but that is what she thought, her and several others who had operations in the seventies and eighties.

The women already in the group were angry too. They were angry that they had no input into the report just published. "It's the same old story. We weren't even spoken to; his word was put before ours." And, of course, the women pointed to the report of the "three wise men" as their proof.

They were angry with themselves too, for believing Neary, for not questioning him. Nicola said she was annoyed at herself "for not screaming at him instead of crying when he told me he removed my womb at nineteen. Before I went to my GP I was still hoping it couldn't be true. But it is. I know that now. There was nothing the matter with me. I am definitely going to a solicitor now."

But most of all they were angry at the suggestion that six months' retraining would solve Dr Neary's problems. The report by Alison O'Connor in *The Irish Times* of 24 April read:

Regarding Dr Neary's future, the Group was of the opinion that the best option was a six-month supervised postgraduate programme where he would have the opportunity to observe colleagues at work in the operating theatre and delivery wards, as well as attending hospital conferences and visiting the laboratory.

That was the greatest insult of all. It resulted in the women regarding this report as a "complete whitewash and not worth bothering about in the end". In fact, they referred to it as "The Whitewash Report".

They were angry too because, despite promises, the women never found out whether their own particular operation fell into the acceptable, unacceptable or doubtful categories. Cathriona said, "I am raging mad at what I've read in the paper – they want him to go back to work. And what about the 'three boyos' that said his work was okay in October? It's saying what happened to us doesn't matter. I am not the same since my operation. I try to look on the bright side and enjoy my two little boys. But I would have liked a little girl. My friend had a girl recently and I am delighted for her but I would love one too. I feel butchered. I think he is off his head, obsessed with sterilising people. He just ranted on at my six-week check up when I asked him about losing my womb. He said he nearly lost his job because the nuns didn't want him to do a tubal ligation. I didn't know what he was talking about. I was numb and he just ranted on."

But Dr Neary was dismayed by the report, we were told by the *Drogheda Independent* on 30 April.

> *"We are not dealing with vast numbers here. Only thirty-nine cases were examined out of literally thousands of cases over his twenty-five years in Our Lady of Lourdes . . . Most of this seventy-page report was praising Dr Neary and his handling of his department. He is a wonderful person, a great doctor and is dismayed by current events," his friend said.*

The women and their families were dismayed too. But matters had moved on. "The main focus of action now is the Medical Council," officials told us. This was what we chose to focus on. But still there was the huge question. Would the Medical Council investigate this man? And if they did, would they do it properly and quickly? Most of the women distrusted the Council. "They will stand up for each other, they always do. Look at what the three wise men did. They defended Neary against us." This was a continuous thorn that created cynicism about the intentions of the Medical Council.

A strange and uncomfortable event happened round this

time too, adding to the women's grief and anger. Several of the women phoned one morning.

Cathriona rang first. "You won't believe what's happened. The hospital has given my name and address to a counselling group in Northern Ireland. I'm invited to a meeting in the Boyne Valley. I think they're trying to wreck our group by setting up another one. I'm not going, for one; I doubt if the others will either. It's shocking."

Nicola was next with the same tale. "They have a nerve doing this. Giving my details out like that. I'm boycotting this. The social work department must have got the details from the contact line and given them out to a counsellor."

"I never trusted the help line," Jenny told me. "Now they're trying to split up our group. It's a divide-and-conquer policy."

Noreen said, "It's the hospital striking back at us."

The women contacted each other and decided they would make their feelings known. They and I felt sorry for the counsellor who had written to all of them, and to other women too no doubt. She was unwittingly caught in the middle. She was in all likelihood unaware of the developing group we had.

I phoned the social work department in the hospital to see what was going on. After several unsuccessful tries I eventually spoke to a social worker. I explained that I was ringing on behalf of the patients in our group. "They are really hurt about this letter. They feel it is an attempt to disrupt their group. They have been working together for months with Dr Tony O'Sullivan and me. Now their confidentiality has been breached by the release of their details to outsiders. They didn't give their permission for this."

"I never heard of your group," the woman at the end of

the phone said. Her voice was jumpy, as if my words or the telephone receiver had given her a sort of electric shock.

I phoned Jim Reilly in the NEHB. This had the potential to derail our fledgling group. Perhaps that was the intention.

"What's happening?" I asked. "The women believe the social work department are setting up an alternative group. They think it is an attempt to divide and conquer. I spoke to this social worker and she tells me she knows nothing about our group. She never heard of us."

"She must have spent the last six months on Mars then," he said.

"Is this a solo by the social work department?" I asked Jim – meaning, was he or the NEHB involved?

"This is the very first I've heard of this."

I was reassured, temporarily at least.

The women themselves were determined not to be undermined by what they saw as an attempt to destroy what they were creating. They wanted to heal themselves and one another. They felt that other hurt women should be told our contact details and left to make up their minds as to whether to get in touch or not. United, they were stronger and better able to support one another.

One of the women accepted the invitation to the "alternative meeting". She told the seventeen women and the counsellor of the existing group. Next morning, I heard of the distress of a young blonde girl, no more than nineteen or twenty, who came with her mother. She ran out of the meeting at one point, such was her distress. I heard also of a midwife at the hospital whose womb had been removed by Neary.

I spoke to Tony, as I was worried by these developments.

"The women's feelings must prevail," he said. "I will explain things to the counsellor."

The counsellor phoned me and suggested we meet for coffee to iron out the problems. In the end everyone agreed that she would continue to counsel the women, both individually and in small groups. The original group would continue to welcome new members into a stronger, united group. They were wounded healers who knew that to heal themselves, they must heal each other too. And the counsellor would help with this, as other counsellors were already doing. In the end it all worked out to the advantage of our group.

This is how our numbers swelled in the late spring and early summer of 1999 and how Cathriona, Nicola and the rest of the initial group met Niamh (the young blonde girl), her mother Helen, Teresa and several others for the first time.

The summer of 1999 was a difficult one. We were making a jigsaw with no idea of the picture the pieces would build. Lots of facts were in the frame, but what did they mean? Each woman had a different explanation if she had one at all.

By midsummer over fifty women had been in touch. Each needed help to find out about her operation. Some too had queries about gynaecological surgery. All were, as Judge Harding Clark would later say, "sound women with supportive spouses". They were bank officials, teachers, nurses, stay-at-home mothers, doctors' office managers, even, very sadly, childminders. They were everywoman. They were a cross-section of women from the north-east of this country, from Cavan, north Dublin, Westmeath, Monaghan, Louth and Meath.

At the meetings, we often talked until one in the morning, overstaying our welcome in the Boyne Valley. They never seemed to mind. Tony provided what reassurance he could. I listened and got to know each couple as friends. I was always struck by the quiet heroism of the men, how they sat by their wives, sometimes coming for them because the women were afraid to come themselves. The men at our meetings were wonderful to their wives. They worried about them, supported them, drove them places, shouldered the bad news when it came, despite knowing that their families too were cut short. They walked hand-in-hand with their wives, taking a back seat when appropriate. They just knew what to do.

One lovely man told me his young wife turned into an old woman overnight after what happened to her. He was now worried that it was all coming back to them again.

"He is an animal, that man," he said with passion. "We have no trust in doctors now. We don't go to them at all."

In May the NEHB told us that experts from Britain were travelling to Drogheda to start the look back into Neary's practice. Women signed consent forms to have the result in their case forwarded to them from the "Whitewash Report".

The NEHB were inundated with women looking for their files and it soon became clear that some could not be found. Ambrose McLoughlin wrote:

I do understand that records of a small number of patients have been unable to be located despite the best efforts of hospital management and staff. In

69

> *light of the failure to locate some records I have*
> *asked an independent company to immediately carry*
> *out a document audit and following this audit I*
> *would expect that all of the missing records should*
> *be accounted for.*

Distrust of the hospital and the help line grew. Some women suspected someone of breaching their confidentiality earlier and now wondered if the same person enabled the removal of their files too. They wondered about the nurses, the midwives, clerical staff, doctors too. They believed they must have known what was happening at the unit. Over and over they asked: "How could this happen without them knowing?" They talked too of the many real kindnesses the nurses and midwives showed to them while they were having their baby and after, and this increased the hurt and confusion.

When Cathriona was taking her new baby home, a young nurse had commented, "Maybe this wouldn't have happened to you if we looked after you better." Cathriona knew she had real concern and caring in her tone.

In June, a small number of the women, clients of Hugh Thornton, one of the solicitors involved, went to Galway to consult Dr Eamon O'Dwyer, a Galway obstetrician, about the need for their caesarean hysterectomy. Hugh arranged it. We were very anxious about this trip, not knowing what to expect, what to hope for. What if we were wrong? Dr O'Dwyer was a former teacher of Neary.

When Cathriona rang to tell me Dr O'Dwyer's opinion, "unnecessary" was the only word she used.

"What?"

"Yes, he looked at my files, put his head in his hands and said I did not need a hysterectomy. I don't think he could believe I was so young. He said what happened to me was tragic." She added, "We couldn't find the house but we ran into Clodagh and her husband going to Dr O'Dwyer. We followed them. Afterwards we met up in Ballinasloe for a meal and he told her the same. She didn't need her womb taken out either. Shocking, isn't it?"

Later that month a third woman rang. She had heard the same terrible news from Dr O'Dwyer.

In July Tony arranged for the Master of the Coombe Women's Hospital in Dublin, Dr Sean Daly, to come to talk to the group about caesarean hysterectomy. He was a quiet-spoken, kind man. He told the women of the small number of such operations carried out in his hospital, two or three a year at most in a much larger centre. He told them of its role in saving lives. The women liked Dr Daly.

It was Niamh and her mother Helen's first meeting. Niamh was just twenty years old and one of the last to be operated on by Neary. It was her plight that caused the midwives to tell of their concerns. Next day Helen rang. She was grateful to Dr Daly and Tony. "Last night was great. I never heard two doctors speak so frankly. People need to be believed. I felt relieved coming home, but feel a fool that we were told so many lies. Neary told us she was dying. And I recommended Neary to Niamh because he delivered her twenty years ago."

In August we arranged for a meeting to introduce the women to a number of solicitors who would advise them legally. And still the numbers were growing, as were the number of missing files. Three solicitors – Colm MacGeehin, Hugh Thornton and Mary O'Neill – attended with a number of barristers. After this meeting, most women consulted one or other of these solicitors. Others had their own family solicitor and preferred to take advice from them. In general, the solicitors would use Irish experts like Prof. John Bonnar, Dr Mary Wingfield, Dr Peter Lenehan and Dr Eamon O'Dwyer. They also received opinions from British-based experts such as Dr Richard Porter and Dr Roger Clements.

At this meeting, the solicitors suggested to the women that they may have felt isolated until now and may have suppressed memories of what had happened to them in Drogheda. Isolation and suppressed memory were very common in medical negligence as, until recently, there was little awareness of patients' rights. Most people believed there was nothing that could be done. They were advised that consent was likely to be a major issue in many Drogheda cases. Many women assumed that the doctor knew best and that there must have been a medical reason for their operation. But now they began to question what they had previously believed was a sound diagnosis and surgical treatment.

They were told it was usually necessary to issue a court summons within three years of the event but that, in relation to Drogheda, the delay in bringing the case could be explained and that this explanation was likely to be accepted by the courts.

Patients often bring a legal case firstly to help in establishing what happened to them and if anyone was responsible for any damage they suffered. Secondly, in order to feel at peace with themselves, they may need a public declaration of the wrong done. Thirdly, people may believe that amends should be made for the wrong. As medical people cannot undo the wrong, financial compensation is the only avenue of restitution open to them. Fourthly, if medical people were negligent, then patients often need to have them identified, have their actions judged by an independent body and have them held accountable. The women themselves had a fifth objective: to prevent a recurrence of their experience for other patients.

The solicitors told the women that they would take cases on a no-win, no-fee basis, but they would be liable for the costs of the other side should they lose. However, each case would have to be judged on its own merits. No case would be pursued unless the medical reports supported a claim of negligence. They reassured them that it looked like many women had strong cases, as the first cases coming back indicated quite shocking negligence.

The solicitors also told the women that a medical negligence action was a long, drawn-out process and would take a considerable amount of time. However, the stress, which is usually considerable, would be lessened if they trusted their legal and medical advisors. In addition, they had each other to provide support during the difficult times, unlike many litigants, who are often alone.

They were also told of the advantage of crossing the threshold from victim to empowered woman by means of asserting and enforcing their rights.

In August too we received a copy of a letter to the legal advisor to the NEHB from the legal advisors to the IOG's Review Group, Coffey & McMahon Solicitors. It refused to give women the Review Group's view of their own particular operation. It read:

> *The three members of the former Review Group regarding Dr Michael Neary met today to consider the request contained in yours of 11th May 1999 and subsequent representations made directly to the Group by the North Eastern Health Board.*
>
> *Our clients can fully understand the desire of the North Eastern Health Board to deal with all former patients of Dr Neary in as sensitive a manner as possible. Our clients also sympathise with the patients concerned and have no wish to cause any further distress in this difficult situation.*
>
> *Following careful deliberations and having given full consideration to the matter our clients have concluded that neither your request, nor that of the Health Board can be met. Apart from other difficulties which out clients have with complying with the request, the functions of the Review Group at this juncture have ceased. It is also clear that the Terms of Reference of the Group as set out in appendix 1 of their report do not provide for the dissemination of this information.*

From the women's point of view, this was a heartbreak that added insult to injury.

"I loved being pregnant," one woman said, "and now I never will be again but they won't even tell me if there was a need for it."

My mother was taken suddenly ill in late summer and died in mid-September. My memory of this period is scant except to say I got great comfort from the friendship of the women. She died at home in the care of my sister and her family. After the funeral a huge bouquet of lilies arrived at my home. Just as my mother filled my childhood home with the smell of ginger bread, brown bread and currant cake, their scent took over my house, it took over my soul at this time and calmed me.

It was mid-October before I could become involved again. Cathriona and I set about organising a meeting of the women and their families at the request of the NEHB. "The Board would like to meet the women and their families and hear their views" was the simple reason given. We weren't sure how this would go down but we felt it was worth a try. Cathriona felt it was a brave thing for the Health Board to do. It was the first real step for the women to talk to those involved.

Sure enough, there was a huge attendance that night. The Boyne Valley's ballroom was set up in cabaret style as usual. A top table always prepared by the hotel staff but never used by Tony and me was not used by the Health Board that night either. They opted to move chairs down near the small tables around which the families congregated. Tony as usual did the introductions. Jim Reilly, Senior Administrative Officer in the Health Board; Mary Duff, Director of Nursing in the Lourdes Hospital; and Sally Campbell, Assistant Director of Nursing, were the three representatives who braved the storm that November evening.

Jim rose to speak. "The Board wishes to apologise unreservedly for what happened to you in Drogheda. We have come here to listen to your concerns and views." Jim expected anger that night and got it, from the men as well as the women. They asked:

- Did no one notice what was happening to young women there before?

- What had happened to the missing files?

- Why were they not told of the result of the IOG's Report in their individual cases?

- What changes have been made to the unit since to ensure no repetition?

- Who were the three obstetricians who supported Neary?

- What about the Medical Missionaries of Mary? What about the midwives and doctors? Should they not be here too?

- What was happening at the Medical Council?

The need for a full inquiry was underlined at this meeting but the full and unreserved apology was, in the main, accepted, through the anger.

Jim told them that "two midwives raised queries with a legal advisor" and they were taken seriously by the Board. He told them of the Maresh report into their care. The support of the NEHB was again offered in relation to medical reports and counselling. There was a promise to renew their quest for the missing files. He described a chaotic filing system of hundreds of cardboard boxes full of files stored in unused rooms, some of which had been flooded. "Theatre records, pathology records and slides will all be examined to see if they could be of help in particular to women whose files are missing." This turned out to be a very helpful initiative. Slides were sourced and forwarded to pathologists for opinions on the pathology or otherwise of the particular specimen. Women without files could have some small idea if they were sick or at risk.

Jim didn't know the identity of the three Irish obstetricians who supported Neary's practice, nor did he know the contents of their reports, except to say, "They were supportive of the doctor and caused serious anxiety in particular for the two midwives."

"Who are the midwives?" the room wondered.

"They are great women," Jim said. In response, they were told that they had been given a guarantee that their identities would never be revealed.

And of course he could not speak for the nuns or the Medical Council but Neary had been suspended from the Medical Register since February pending a full inquiry.

But most of all, Jim told them that no further caesarean hysterectomy had been performed at the hospital since the removal of Neary almost a year before. This calmed things.

Mary Duff was robustly questioned about what she knew. Sally Campbell sat by her side, silent but in support of her colleague.

"I did not know it was happening," Mary said. "I had no idea." The overwhelming message was that the womb of young woman after young woman was removed unnecessarily and no one noticed.

"How long were you there while Neary was mutilating women?" she was asked.

77

"Four years," she said, "but the maternity unit was separate from the rest of the hospital in that general staff did not visit the unit. It ran itself, even since it was integrated into the main hospital in the early nineties." In other words, it was a no-go area for general nursing staff.

There were no representatives of the maternity unit there that night. That was not lost on the gathering. The doctors and nurses most closely involved were missing. Others were sent out to bear the heat. There was respect for those who came, though no one there knew of the role of Mary Duff in taking the allegations against Neary seriously once they were made known to her. This meeting was the first real engagement with the group and helped enormously in developing trust that this matter would be resolved at some stage, even if that took far too long.

The meeting over, people streamed out of the ballroom and stood around in clusters in the cold damp November air. There was huge disbelief at the denial of knowledge. In truth, no one believed. People tossed the events of the evening around in their heads. They did not seem to want to go home, such was the need to digest what was said.

"An apology from the Health Board is no good to me. It was the nuns who were in charge when it happened to me."

"Where are the nuns? Are they going to come here and answer questions?"

"And where is Neary? He is going about his business as if nothing happened. I see him in Dunnes buying his cat food."

Anger was growing too about the silence from the profession and the Medical Council, not to mention the Minister for Health and the Department. The Council was conducting its own inquiry but the women were never informed of progress. This lack of contact caused great distrust.

In fairness, it should be said that the Council believed that processes and procedures in relation to Fitness to Practise inquiries under the Medical Practitioners Act of 1978 made this very difficult. They had made submissions to the Department to update the legislation and they were awaiting a response. However, the women did not or could not know of this at that stage.

In the weeks that followed, the NEHB sought the help of the pathology department at the Lourdes to find slides for women whose files were missing. We were told this help was forthcoming. All in all, progress was snail-slow, but it was progress all the same.

In the early weeks of the new millennium, at the request of the women, Tony issued a press release making the NEHB's apology public. He called on the Minister for Health Brian Cowen to establish a public inquiry into all aspects of gynaecological and obstetric care over the last twenty years at Our Lady of Lourdes Hospital, Drogheda. *"The women feared a repetition of these events unless lessons were learned from them and unless changes were made to the consultants' contract and other aspects of professional regulation to improve accountability and facilitate disclosure of future concerns by health workers at all levels,"* he wrote.

There was a sense, once the second Christmas had passed, that some order was growing from the chaos and shock of the original disclosures in the media and the ensuing professional reviews. The women were beginning to find their own personal truth, even if in a very painful way. Their emotional strength was growing.

Patient Focus was formally established too. Now the women had a definite, legally constituted organisation to fight for them and make their presence felt in the political sphere.

Part 2

Politicians and Professionals

4

Capturing the Minister

The women were very frustrated at the January and March 2000 meetings. Another painful Christmas had come and gone. The new millennium had dawned but nothing was happening that they were aware of. No one seemed to care. Furthermore, people in the town of Drogheda and surrounding areas seemed not to believe them or show interest in their tragedy. At least, that was what they thought.

Tony wrote to Minister Cowen in January asking for a meeting but received no reply. By March there had been a change of Minister. Micheál Martin was now in charge, but probably learning his way into his job. Nevertheless, a reply should have been received. Was the Minister totally uninterested, did he not believe them, or was he more interested in hiding things? The answer, the women suspected, was probably all three. There was a late winter mood about, a belief that their particular winter would never end if things continued as they were. We talked late, until about half past midnight as at all other meetings, but the mood was pessimistic and self-reproaching.

The long and painful road they were travelling, the battles to get their files, the medical examinations, the facing of legal reports telling tales they did not want to believe, the family difficulties, the new friends made, all of this was forgotten, such was the despondency that evening. Something clearly had to be done.

Tony suggested they write to the new Minister for Health individually as patients. Forget the letter from Patient Focus. It was time now to flood Micheál Martin with their requirements for a public independent inquiry into the hospital. The meeting agreed with him. As many women as possible would write to the Minister, telling him their stories and asking him to meet them. This was their first step in politicisation. But it was no faltering baby step. It was taken calmly and with resolve. There was no ranting here, no hysteria, no whipping up of emotion. Just the determination of hurt women to find out the truth, to protect their daughters in the future, and to obtain justice for themselves in the present. Their difficulties were going to be taken to the Minister, the political parties, local councillors and even to the gates of the Dáil, if necessary. They had been passive, good little girls for too long, they thought; now they were to become women with a purpose. And so they did.

Over the next few weeks, many women wrote to the Minister. This was hard for everyone. It was April before the acknowledgements started to arrive on their mats in the form of a holding letter from Bernard O'Shea, the Minister's private secretary. A substantive reply arrived in May. Its message? "This is a matter in the first instance for the NEHB."

The women were mad after all the letter writing, after all the passion, the effort to explain the enormity of what had happened. Still no one was listening, even those charged with the legal responsibility for the care of the nation's health. Iseult, a woman always so articulate and courageous, was "incandescent with rage". She reminded me of a Celtic queen with her dark curly hair, a warrior woman of passion like Queen Maeve from a Jim Fitzpatrick print, a small but passionate woman who knows right from wrong and will defend it.

To me, however, it was no surprise. The civil service was being the civil service, acting true to form. There was no point in letting some civil servant put you off. They would want to protect their minister from bad publicity. I felt sure that if we got past the front guard we would be okay. I decided to ring Bernard O'Shea.

This turned out to be an even more frustrating process than I imagined. I was fobbed off, left on hold, told to ring back tomorrow over and over. I decided to ring each morning for a number of mornings and never succeeded in speaking to the same person twice. Bernard O'Shea was either not at his desk, unavailable or so important he could not speak to me, and this despite telling everyone I spoke to that I wanted to talk to him about setting up a meeting with the Minister and a number of young women whose wombs were unnecessarily removed by a Drogheda obstetrician. I left my phone number each day and waited until the next day, when I would begin the whole rigmarole again. My calls were never returned.

Eventually I was so annoyed I went to my computer and typed out the following note:

8/5/00

Dear Mr O'Shea

I refer to a letter Dr Tony O'Sullivan received from you dated 18/4/00 concerning the practice of obstetrics in Our Lady of Lourdes Hospital. Dr O'Sullivan and I speak for fifty women and their families. It is eighteen months now since news of this particular medical tragedy and indeed serious scandal broke. The women have asked us to arrange a meeting for them with the Minister for Health to inform him firsthand of how they have been damaged. Some were as young as eighteen when, it appears, they had their wombs removed unnecessarily as they were giving birth by caesarean section.

They feel that they are being ignored by the Department of Health. A letter to Minister Cowen in January from Patient Focus was not even acknowledged. Further letters from the women themselves and from Patient Focus have been merely acknowledged with no follow-on reply. The women say these acknowledgements are not worth the stamps used unless followed up with a thoughtful reply and a meeting with the Minister.

On a daily basis I hear them express the view that nothing has been learned from the Blood Board scandals in terms of how to treat people damaged by health care. They say injured people are still abandoned, treated as nuisances, told as little as possible, while everyone responsible closes their eyes, hopes they will go away.

I rang the Minister's office this morning and was advised that you were not available to talk to me. It was suggested I ring back tomorrow when I could talk to Veronica, not you. I was very worried and disappointed by the lack of urgency with which my request was treated.

Some matters are so profoundly wrong that it is required of us all to do what is necessary to resolve them. Unfortunately this is one of these issues. These women and their families have been incredibly patient. They deserve to have their terrible stories listened to by the person responsible for the administration of health care. They deserve to meet the Minister for Health as a matter of urgency. I'm sure Minister Martin will not let them down as others have done.

Hoping to hear from you very soon indeed.

Sheila O Connor

I rang up the department again and asked for Bernard O'Shea's fax number. Within an hour, my fax was sent. And within the hour, I received a phone call.

"Sheila. This is Agnes Twomey. I'm phoning on behalf of Bernard O'Shea. We got your fax and it is on Bernard's desk. He will talk to the Minister about it and I will be back to you as soon as possible."

"Oh, that's great. How long do you expect that to take?"

"I should be back in about forty-eight hours."

Some movement at last.

On a fine May day we met the Minister for Health and Children.

Niamh, Nicola, Cathriona, Jenny, Iseult and I met at lunchtime. We laughed nervously as we huddled round a small table in Buswell's Hotel, across the road from Leinster House. We had sandwiches and pots of tea and coffee. We tried to whisper but the nerves were taut and it was hard to do. Others should not hear the nature of our mission.

The questions flew about. What would we say? Who would talk? How many would be there with him?

Iseult is particularly annoyed. "We will talk about his insulting letters," she says, referring to the letters from Bernard O'Shea.

I rooted in my bag for a piece of paper. "We need to write an agenda. Have some general idea of what we will say." I started to scribble words:

- *Introduce ourselves*
- *Make general statement – about physical, emotional and sexual abuse by Neary over long period*
- *Impossible that other professionals didn't know*
- *Tribunal of Inquiry*
- *Tribunal of Compensation*
- *Legislative change to Medical Council*
- *Invite to meet the big group*

This was written on a dodgy political pamphlet I found in my bag – no doubt handed to me in a pub somewhere and not cleared out. But it had its uses that day. "We can't take that out at the meeting," I said, looking at the state of it. "We will just have to operate from memory. But at least we know the main points to make."

We piled into a people carrier taxi to take us to the Minister's office. In Hawkins House, we waited for the Minister in a small meeting room, sitting around a long table that almost filled the room. The Minister swept in with his entourage. He was dressed in his shirtsleeves because of the heat.

I introduced us after the Minister asked: "Which of you is Sheila O Connor?" He apologised for the difficulty in making contact. He knows it is hard to get through. We made light of it.

Then the women told their stories. Niamh, Nicola, Cathriona, Jenny, Iseult. We really hadn't planned this but it happened. Gobnait O'Connell, the Minister's personal advisor, looked shocked at the other side of the table and cried softly. Iseult had her say about the letter. She read the offending phrase: "This is a matter in the first instance for the NEHB."

"Who wrote this?" the Minister asked. An assistant principal in the department stated that she had.

"I am sorry," said the Minister. He looked like he meant it.

He agreed to come and meet the bigger group in Drogheda during July. It would be a private meeting with no media in attendance.

"Exchange phone numbers," he said to an official. "Make sure there is a contact number for people." And she did.

The women were impressed that he agreed to come to Drogheda, but were in bits after laying grief bare to strangers. Why did this have to be so hard?

Over the next six weeks we repeated this exercise with the opposition leader John Bruton and his health spokesperson, Gay Mitchell. We were gently received there too.

On 19 July 2000, another fine summer's evening, Minister for Health Micheál Martin travelled to the Boyne Valley Hotel in Drogheda to meet the women and their families. Tony and I met him and Gobnait when they arrived at the hotel foyer.

"It makes it much easier that Tony is involved," the Minister said, referring to the fact that he was a doctor and nodding in his direction.

"It's easier for the women too," I said.

The women really appreciated the Minister's visit and said so. They marvelled at how lightly government travelled – one black car at the hotel door. He promised to do what he could that evening but said his hands were tied until the Medical Council reached a decision. "I am precluded from interfering in how they conduct their affairs. They refused to provide me with any information at all," he told a full ballroom of about a hundred people seated around small tables. He circulated among them and spoke to most.

Cathriona had conducted a survey of the women to give him so that he could have a more personal account of the damage Neary perpetrated. She handed it to Gobnait for safe keeping. Cathriona had spent a month working in the evenings putting it together. She typed it to make it easy for him to read. It was more a collection of personal testimonies than a survey. It had a sacred feel at the time and still does.

"A very bad dream I can't wake up from. I cry at inappropriate places and times," was how one young victim described her feelings. She was one of the last of his victims and was told in the theatre as he was performing the surgery. She begged him not to do it. "After the operation the hospital tiptoed round me . . . and sent a social worker to talk to me. He [Neary] was happy at my post-natal check up, complimented me on my looks and was very chatty, talking about the other women's lives he saved. I hate myself for going to him, being lied to, and my usual easy-going trusting attitude to life is gone."

A young victim from the early eighties wrote: "He told me at my six-week check up. I had no idea till then. I couldn't believe what I was hearing. I was only twenty-six years old. My womb was gone. It was my second child. I wanted four or five. He said I had a ruptured womb, uncontrollable bleeding, it was a matter of life and death. I should be grateful to him for saving my life and if my husband wanted to adopt he would put in a good word for me. When I rang the hospital looking for my notes recently, they would not give me any straight answers. They gave me the impression that it was a long time ago and I should have forgotten about it by now, but I ignored them. It broke up our marriage for a while. I was depressed for a number of years and my husband fell to pieces, but we worked hard at our marriage, thank God. I always knew that Neary did me wrong. I carried this knowing all these years. It was a relief to know I was right when the truth came out. I tried to do something about it at the time, went to a solicitor, but I got nowhere. An ordinary person couldn't sue a doctor, no matter what he did."

Another woman asked: "How could something of this magnitude go on for so long unreported? Where were the nuns, the nurses, the other professional people who must have been aware of the huge problems this man had? We know consultants adopt god-like attitudes and if they are doing their work professionally one could almost forgive them because ultimately good will come of it. But when they are incompetent and are savaging their patients physically and mentally!! What procedures are in place to protect the patient's rights? When patients are ill they are not in a position to think clearly or to protect their rights. All of the hospital personnel who facilitated this man in his reign of terror should be made to accept their share of the blame for the lives this man has destroyed. Consultants should be regularly tested and appraised by an independent body. The Inquiry that initially found that all this man needed was an update in his skills should be very seriously monitored in its future decisions. The mothers of Ireland have had to endure the hepatitis C scandal and the organs scandal. The knowledge that the remains of their babies have been lying in bottles on the shelves of hospitals or, worse still, thrown out with the refuse or incinerated, is an unmerciful burden for bereaved parents. If the case we are making to the Minister for Health and Children prevents one other person being abused and assaulted by the medical profession, then the terror, trauma and heartache I have experienced since my dealings with this man will be worthwhile."

The very sad voice of a young woman comes through in the following: "He told me I had a muscle defect, uncontrollable bleeding; it was a matter of life and death. I was told in theatre just before it was performed. At my six-week check up he was very unsympathetic. He told me I was lucky to be alive and gave me a crazy reason as to why it happened. The hospital didn't seem to care. They didn't treat it as a serious situation. It wasn't talked about. I was offered no counselling, just handed a book to read about hysterectomy; none of it related to my case. Physically I am okay but emotionally I will never get over the fact of not being able to have more children. I feel robbed of my femininity. I hate doctors. I feel empty and incomplete. I feel I have been lied to and cheated on. I don't know what normal is any more. This was my first pregnancy, and I am heartbroken to say my only one."

That night women told the Minister they have an enormous fear of doctors. They do not trust them now. They avoid going to them. They mentioned the support that the three Irish doctors gave Neary. They doubted the commitment of the Medical Council to investigate one of their own; to date nothing had been heard from them. Three complaints had not even been acknowledged after eighteen months. How could that inspire trust? When was their inquiry going to happen? Was it ever going to happen? What more did they need? How much longer would it take? The women cited how the IOG review group behaved, interviewing Neary but not them. They wouldn't tell them if their own particular operation was necessary. They took their files without asking their permission. They looked only at cases from 1992 to 1998. They knew, of course, that this was just the tip of the iceberg. Neary had been at it since 1978, they knew for certain. In fact, four women who were operated on that year were in the room. They knew what they knew, they told the Minister. And worst of all, they said, Neary could return to work after some training.

"How could people like that be trusted?" they asked that summer night.

They sought Gobnait out too and told her their stories. They felt she listened.

Micheál Martin promised to come back to them in September with news of the timeframe for the Medical Council Inquiry. No other specific promises were made by the Minister at the meeting.

5

Ethics and Etiquette

In September I phoned Catherine Bannon, one of the civil servants dealing with the matter in the Department. I told her that enormous goodwill had been built up as a result of Micheál Martin's visit to Drogheda. I did not want this to dissolve. We were planning to have a further meeting at the end of September and we expected to have news of developments. Catherine knew of none and advised me to write to the Minister. I wrote on 11 September reminding him of his commitment to the women to get back to them by September concerning the issues raised at the July meeting.

Gobnait O'Connell called me and asked me to delay the meeting until October; there may be substantive news then. She asked me to tell the women that the Minister found the meeting very helpful in understanding the issues involved. She would ring in the first week of October with news.

That same week Dr Roger Clements came to Ireland to examine at least nine of the women and prepare medico-legal reports, at the request of their solicitor Hugh Thornton. All had had caesarean hysterectomies. This was very traumatic for the women. In the week following I spoke to several of the women. Dr Clements had been upset by what he found. None of the women he examined needed their operation in his view. This mood was taken on board by the women.

Cathriona told me what Clements had said to her. "He wouldn't speculate further about what was going on in Neary's mind."

Clements alleged collusion with other members of staff, at least in relation to not revealing what had happened and deliberate false recording of events. (It should be noted that the Lourdes Hospital Inquiry made no finding of collusion.)

Dr Clements' medical opinion was so devastating that I wrote another letter to the Minister on 16 September.

Dear Mr Martin,

Over the last couple of days several of the women in our group have consulted an obstetrician concerning his opinion as to the quality of the care they received in Our Lady of Lourdes Hospital. I have spent some time talking to them after their visits. The opinions they received back up reports already obtained from other obstetricians.

The nature of the medical details emerging are terrifying. It is difficult not to conclude that the truth unfolding surpasses in extent and depravity even the most notorious sexual assault cases that have been tried in our courts in recent times. It appears from these reports that none of it could have happened over such a long period without the knowledge and collusion of other members of staff, including medical and nursing personnel. Most worryingly, why were complaints by individual patients ignored and why did it take young newly recruited staff to express concern to a non-health care professional, outside the hospital, before any action was taken?

All of the women and their partners are even more insistent now on the need for a public and independent inquiry as a minimum political reaction at this stage. They say they can keep quiet no longer. The young couple whose baby died after an "emergency" caesarean hysterectomy at nineteen years has a right to demand and obtain answers to these truly terrible questions.

I look forward to hearing from you as a matter of urgency.

Yours sincerely,
Sheila O Connor.

Writing this letter worried me. I sought legal opinion. "It is a fair summary of what the doctor said to the women." Hugh Thornton was in shock about what his English expert was telling him he found.

This young country gentleman solicitor was for once almost speechless. The adhesive quality of guilt was sticking to him. "Imagine, this man's victims are going in and out of my office. I feel guilty that I defended the hospital in the past and didn't believe when people described medical treatment

as assault, that they thought a doctor should be in jail."
Then he said, "It is up to you to engage in the political and
media aspects of this to make sure it never happens again. To
make sure people find out. Who would believe this was
going on?" I could almost see his head shake in astonishment
across the phone.

I posted my letter.

Gobnait died outside Kinnegad on 19 September. That
evening as I drove my daughter Aideen home from school,
AA Roadwatch warned of the traffic build-up in the
Kinnegad area because of a very bad accident. Aideen was
alone with me that day, no friends bumming a lift for once.

"How was school today?"

For some reason she wanted to talk.

"My teacher said today that we have the best health
service in the world."

"Ours is probably as good as most but that doesn't mean
there's not lots wrong with it," I said.

"I couldn't say in his class that they weren't nice to
Granny."

"We looked after her well, didn't we?" I said.

"I know, but the nurses weren't that nice. They left her
sitting on chairs all the time. She wasn't happy there."

"Everyone needs a minder when they're in hospital and
we brought her home, didn't we? Why couldn't you say that
in class, anyway?"

"Everyone would think I was weird," she said. "The
essay I wrote about the work you do . . . I said you help
people hurt by doctors and my teacher put a line under it
and a question mark. She thought I said it wrong."

"That doesn't mean she wouldn't understand if you explained," I said. "After all, the essay was in Irish and she probably thought you got it upside down. Your Irish could do with some improvement and maybe that's what she's bothered about."

"I'm in the highest Irish class."

The subject was changed. Aideen too was going through a type of bereavement coming up to her Granny's first anniversary.

The next morning, the 7.30 news included a very distressing story. Gobnait O'Connell was driving back from Tullamore where the Minister for Health was unveiling his vision of health care for the next ten years. Her car hit a coach head on.

I barely knew her. Most of the women, except for the small number who went to meet the Minister, had met her just once. Yet my phone started to ring at 7.50. They had placed their faith in Gobnait's energy and in Gobnait's heart. They asked me to write to the Minister and tell him of their sorrow. They wanted to send flowers to the funeral of a woman they had met once, a woman they saw as an ally. They had handed over their stories in a binder for safe-keeping, for Gobnait's eyes and the Minister's eyes only.

I did as they all wanted. It was easy. That day the previous year had been the last day of my mother's life too. I thought of Gobnait's mother. For days the phone calls kept coming. Gobnait was their trusted route to the truth coming out.

I heard nothing about my letters to the Minister until 11 October, when a principal officer in the Secondary Care Unit rang to confirm receipt of my letter and to say it was receiving attention at the very highest level in the Department. I told him that the lack of news from the Department was making the women lose faith and they would appreciate a response soon. His reply was that the purpose of his phone call was merely to acknowledge receipt of my letter. But he hoped I would receive one shortly. I never received a reply.

A few days later, one of the women phoned. "I just want to tell you that the night he did my hysterectomy, he did two that night."

"What! Are you sure?"

"Positive. It was a woman I knew. She'd just had her baby. We spoke to each other, compared notes. It's definitely true."

I rang Tony. "That should have rung alarm bells for the staff," he said, "just as it's doing for us."

Other staff must have known. I thought of the woman who told me of how her doctor, who was away at the time of "the emergency", avoided contact with her after Neary removed her womb. Neary, of course, gallantly stood in for him – saved the day, saved her life, he would say. But the other doctor had reddened when he'd heard.

Later, after one of our meetings, another woman and her husband talked to Tony and me about the birth of her first and only baby. "My legs were in stirrups and he was so rough. Dr Neary spread them further, forced them apart with his elbows." She moved her elbows out and back in demonstration and remembering. "To me they were like the movements of a rugby player breaking a scrum to get the ball. I refused to speak to him afterwards. I would not speak to him when he came on his rounds, I felt so badly. So hurt and humiliated."

"Normal obstetricians do not behave like that," I said.
"Normal human beings don't," added Tony.

Nicola visited her GP after receiving her legal report from Dr Clements.

"He won't accept Neary did it deliberately. He still thinks he was just nervous," she said. She was very upset when she received the report. "I read it three times before I could take it all in. Then I put it on top of the wardrobe so I would not come across it by accident. I am not going to let him destroy me again. He has taken everything anyway. He can take no more."

In the spring of 2000, I was recommended for appointment as patient advocate, by Mary Duff, Director of Nursing at the Lourdes Hospital, to the Curriculum Development Committee for Midwifery (Direct Entry). This was an interesting collaborative venture by Trinity College, the Rotunda and Our Lady of Lourdes Hospital to train mature women who are not nurses as midwives. A shortage of midwives precipitated this venture. The fourth meeting of the committee was to be held in the boardroom of the Rotunda, the oldest maternity hospital in Ireland.

The women who were former patients of Neary believed strongly that the midwives needed to hear their stories. They were disappointed that no one from the maternity unit had come to the meeting in November 1999 when the health board had apologised. They wanted to break this lack of engagement. I thought I might use my position on the development committee to encourage this.

Earlier, I had tried to raise the possibility of members of our group talking to the student midwives. I had been invited to a reception in the Atrium, Trinity College, on a sultry summer's evening, to celebrate the start of the course. We stood around drinking wine in light summer finery. I recognised a familiar face, a senior midwife recently recruited to the Drogheda hospital, totally free of responsibility for previous practices. We had met before. I considered her a lovely woman, someone with the best interests of birthing women at heart, someone who would be desperate to prevent brutality in the labour ward and mutilation in the delivery room.

Initial small talk used up, I said, "Maybe at some point a few women from the support group could talk of their personal experiences to the students."

She blushed and there was alarm in her eyes. She moved out of earshot and lowered her head to mine in case anyone else should overhear us.

"Oh no," she said. "That would really hurt the staff."

I was taken aback. It was as if I had behaved obscenely in polite company. After this, I left as soon as I thought etiquette allowed.

I decided to go to the October meeting in the Rotunda and try again. I looked around the boardroom. A rich vibrant blue and yellow carpet covered polished wooden floors. The design was large and floral. An impressive wooden table rested in the room's centre. The walls were covered in portraits of important-looking men, some in robes, men I took to be past Masters of the Rotunda. *In the boardroom of the birthing house only men are honoured, like popes in the Vatican*, I thought, but did not say. I had never noticed all this before. I had never taken in the detail of the physical surroundings.

As usual, the meeting was very well organised. The

convenor had everything at her fingertips. She managed this committee wonderfully, always ordered, polite, dedicated. She was dressed in a soft linen-type cream dress and loose jacket. She had worn this at the reception in Trinity.

They were formidable women in the very best sense. I both envied them and felt sad for them. Envy, because if you assist a birthing woman, the glory must rub off on you somehow. Once a woman has given birth under her own steam, she thinks she can do anything. Sad, because the over-use of medicine, in Drogheda, had taken this wondrousness from them.

Midwives walked several footsteps behind the doctor instead of out front with the woman giving birth. They should be cross, but they were not. They did not wish, or were afraid, to take on board the implications of midwifery being the profession they professed it to be. This was made very clear to me now when I again suggested that some of the women in our group come and speak to the committee, a suggestion much watered-down from my original one, that they speak to the student midwives.

"We will think about it," the convenor said. Think about it. What was there to think about? Where was the ethics in refusing to listen to people damaged by the practices of a member of an allied profession, one you supported, one that influenced the practice of your own profession?

It is the antithesis of what professionalism should be. The supremacy of etiquette over ethics in midwifery training. That's what happened in Drogheda, I thought.

Róisín's Story

Róisín and Conor come from Carrickmacross, County Monaghan, a town with a long and rich tradition of lace-making, a tradition resurrected by the St Louis nuns in the nineteenth century. This delicate and complex lace is still made there today. Róisín works in commerce and finance, but I can easily imagine a lace-maker ancestor. I can see Róisín wearing lace.

Róisín was the first of our group to tell her story to the members of the Fitness to Practise Committee of the Medical Council in its Inquiry into Michael Neary. We arrived early on the morning of 16 October 2000. We waited upstairs in the offices of the Medical Council in Portobello. We were unsure of everything. But Róisín looked calm. She had travelled there by the early morning bus with Noreen. All the women came without their husbands. This was the first time I'd seen Róisín without Conor.

She looked composed, I thought, this mother of two small boys with her gentle voice. The first time I met her, about eighteen months earlier, she spoke softly of her delight in them. Róisín always speaks gently. I left her company with the feeling that, despite everything, there is good in the world. Now she was to tell her story to the Medical Council.

With a clear objective she decided, "I have to tell my story. If I don't, I am like the people in the hospital who didn't tell. I cannot be like that. It happened to my friend too. We thought it was because of something we did that this happened. Or we thought it was maybe something in our work. In the office machinery or something." Róisín, like the rest of the women, was willing to suffer to tell their story. And suffer she did. She had to wait for five hours before she could tell her story, cooped up in a small box-like room, waiting to tell the truth.

She told the committee the story she had hinted at to me. I knew not to go any further. She represents the women to me. In their company, her extraordinary story is ordinary.

In 1994 she had a trouble-free pregnancy with her second baby and Michael Neary was her doctor. Because she'd had a section with her first baby, she understood when he suggested a section this time, as it would save her going into labour. She went into hospital the night before. "I hadn't made up my mind about an epidural or to be put out for the operation," she told the committee. "The anaesthetist came and went into the pros and cons. I decided to have an epidural."

The section was due at ten o'clock, then postponed until twelve. "Dr Neary put his nose in the door to check I was okay, and said the operation would go ahead at twelve noon."

Róisín's husband would have liked to have been there when her baby was born. "I think he asked on the way down but they said no. That was as far as he could go," she explained.

"The anaesthetist gave me an injection. Dr Neary came in . . . Things started to move after that. It was not long before my baby was born." A young nurse held Róisín's hand during the operation to deliver her baby.

"When my baby was born, Dr Neary said the cord was tight round his neck. He came out crying his eyes out, a fine healthy baby. Then they showed me the baby. I was overjoyed. They took him away. I was still holding the nurse's hand. I was overjoyed with delight in the baby."

Then Dr Neary said her womb wasn't contracting.

"I didn't hold the baby. They put him beside me. I kissed him. It was then it was said that my womb was not contracting," Róisín continued. "In my joy after having the baby I thought that it will be fine in a minute. I had a healthy baby boy. I was not overly concerned. Then there was silence for about twenty seconds. Everyone was quiet, no one said anything. I was not aware of anything untoward happening to me. I was holding the nurse's hand. It struck me suddenly; I had a friend who had a hysterectomy some time previously. Suddenly it hit me. I said to the nurse, 'He wouldn't take it out.' Then Dr Neary said, 'It has to come out.'"

There was no discussion.

"It happened that quickly. They set to work straight away, I had no more say in the matter." It was two to three minutes between when Róisín's baby was born and when they set to work. "They started to work down on my womb and the shock hit me suddenly, that is it. I wouldn't have any

more children. My family is cut short. I started to wish my little boy was a little girl. I started to give out to myself. I had a healthy baby and should not be thinking like that. Then I consoled myself, I would adopt two little girls. All these things were going through my head like lightning. Next thing I could feel them working in my stomach, trying to take out the womb. I started to feel very sick. I was holding tight to the nurse's hand and those thoughts were gone then. I was trying to cope with the operation. I was very uncomfortable. I was getting sick . . . They worked quickly and did not talk.

"Next thing, he said, 'We are out of danger.' Obviously he had taken out the womb." At this stage they started to talk. Neary told Róisín that he had seen this problem before. "He reckoned it was caused by my mother . . . when she wanted to stop breastfeeding."

There was no sense of emergency, she told the hearing. "They were quiet. All he said was the womb wasn't contracting. Then they set to work. No one said anything. Then he said we were out of the danger area. He chatted casually, easily, not like a panic at all."

It was 1.10 when Róisín went out to recovery, her baby delivered and womb removed in this short period of time. Róisín believed it was to save her life.

"When I came out I was crying my eyes out. There was a midwife and she said Dr Neary had to do that to save your life. I did not doubt her. I thought that was correct, but I wasn't going to stop crying anyway. I nodded in agreement as I was crying. She said, 'Do you want me to tell your husband?' I shook my head and said, 'I will tell him myself.' That is all the dealings I had in the recovery room."

Next evening, Dr Neary came in to see her and said, "Oh pasty, pasty," and pulled down her eyelids. He arranged for her to receive two pints of blood the day after her baby was born.

A couple of days later, Neary sat down at Róisín's bed, quite casually. Her husband was there. It was the speed with which she was losing blood, he told them. He told them too about a twenty-year-old girl whose womb he had to remove. "I didn't want to do it," he said, but he had to in the end.

"When he talked about the other girl I felt he deliberated about it for hours. It seemed there was consideration. Mine happened so quickly," Róisín said. Róisín got no blood during her operation.

Róisín and her husband were very sad about the hysterectomy. They would have liked more children. They enquired about adoption, but always felt the operation was necessary to save her life.

Róisín's operation was not necessary. She was the first of eleven women who gave evidence to that committee over the course of that week. Dr Neary was found guilty of professional misconduct in Róisín's case.

6

In Lynn House

Irish doctors regulate themselves. The statutory body that regulates medical practice in Ireland is the Medical Council. Sometimes doctors are accused of wrongdoing. In such cases a Fitness to Practise committee is formed. This is a subcommittee of the Council. A preliminary hearing is conducted to see if there is a prima facie case to be answered on the basis of the evidence before the committee.

In 2000, of the twenty-five members of the Council, four were lay members; the remainder were doctors. The Council appoints a barrister to present its case to the committee. The doctor appoints a barrister to represent him or her, paid for by the insurance company.

In 2000, Council hearings were almost always held behind closed doors. The patient was a witness, with no right to legal representation. When giving evidence, they were permitted to be accompanied by a family member as a general rule. Often they gave evidence alone.

This is what happened in the case of Michael Neary. The Fitness to Practise committee decided on 6 June 2000 that Michael Neary had a case to answer. This was fifteen months after he was suspended from the medical register by the High Court on the Council's recommendation. The full hearing began on 16 October 2000 in the offices of the Council, Lynn House in Portobello, Dublin city. This was the first opportunity the women had to tell their stories.

In Lynn House they were uncomfortable with patients around. They didn't know what to do with them. To start with, when they invited the women to give evidence at a Fitness to Practise hearing, they warned them of the absolute confidentiality of the proceedings. A letter told them they were not to talk to anyone about the hearing. The implication was that there would be trouble if they broke this rule. There was the feeling of an underlying threat rather than an actual one. The women felt that some dastardly deed would befall them if they spoke, much like what happens in hospitals when people complain. The culture of total secrecy was here too. The Council, the women thought, did not understand the difference between confidentiality and secrecy.

Then the Council waited until the last moment to tell them of the venue for the hearing, lest news got out and there was publicity, I supposed. It was the Friday afternoon of the last working day before the hearing when the women were told it was to be held in Lynn House.

I met Róisín and Noreen early on the first morning of the hearings. We were in a very small room together in Lynn House. They were waiting to be called to give evidence. I was hoping to be allowed to attend the hearing with one of the other women, Nicola. They were aware that Neary was likely to be in the building for the start of the hearing. They were very concerned that they would in all likelihood come face-to-face with him there and wanted company. Meeting Neary was a particular dread for all of the women.

We were unsure of everything. But Róisín and Noreen looked calm. Much calmer than I felt. They had travelled together by the early morning bus. All the women decided to come without their husbands. This was the first time I'd seen Róisín without Conor and Noreen without Martin.

There was a preliminary application by barrister Dr Michael Forde at the request of solicitor Colm MacGeehin for the hearings to be in public. Colm acted on behalf of a number of the women in their civil negligence cases against Neary. They also made allegations of professional misconduct to the Council against him and were to give evidence. I could attend that.

I had breached confidentiality when I spoke to the media and told them of the date and location of the hearing. I had spent the weekend phoning the papers, RTÉ, journalists I have come to know, leaving messages on their voicemails, with colleagues, with their wives, warning them of the confidentiality and respect due, extracting promises that they would not photograph or film the women. They all agreed. They knew the real story would not come for a while yet.

"This will be some story in the end," Aileen O'Meara, a journalist from RTÉ said. I agreed.

Mary Finlay, the barrister on Neary's side, waved a copy of the piece by Fergal Bowers in the *Sunday Independent*. Clearly it proved my unsuitability to sit with the women as they gave their evidence. I went public, broke the golden rule of secrecy. It reminded me of the times when parents and family were not allowed to visit children in hospital; brothers and sisters were forbidden in maternity wards; and husbands could not be with their wives as they laboured or gave birth.

I had to leave as they considered the application that I be allowed to attend with Nicola when she gave her evidence. As I left, I looked Neary in the eye. He looked away before I did. This surprised me. I sat on the stairs waiting as they decided if I could fulfil my promise to Nicola and sit with her as she gave evidence. They decided I could not go in. That was that.

Over the next few days my work involved sitting around, just in case. It involved me drinking lots of coffee in a little coffee shop nearby, reading a Dermot Bolger book, feeding the meter. The coffee was good and the potato and leek soup with fennel bread was even better, but it was a sad wait. And that morning the wait was only starting.

One by one, the women went in to give evidence. Those without family with them were exceptionally allowed have their solicitor with them, for support alone. No news other than the women's version was available of what was transpiring behind the closed door of the hearing room.

Niamh was there to tell her story, along with her mother. They looked more like sisters than mother and daughter. They acted more like sisters too, such is the quality of their friendship. But Helen is Niamh's mother and she carried more pain about this than a sister would. She gasped nervously when Neary came into the coffee shop at lunchtime. He swooped in like an eagle, his collection of solicitors and barristers all dressed in black like undertakers. Except for Mary Finlay. She wore a professional navy skirt suit and white blouse. The coffee shop was small and held about twenty in all.

Niamh went grey. Helen was conducting a vigil, watching her daughter. "This is the hardest thing you will ever have to do in your life," Helen told Niamh.

Trying to be reassuring, knowing words were redundant, I said, "At least you've come face-to-face now. Bear in mind that he has very good reason to be afraid of you. He cannot hurt you more," I added, afraid it was untrue.

We sat and tried to eat our soup. None of us was hungry.

Niamh and Helen waited all day and were not called to give evidence. They would have to come back again the next morning.

Next morning early, Niamh was stuck in traffic. I was amazed that she still wanted me there. I told her we would meet after I was interviewed by Paul Maguire on LMFM. I told him all I could. I was beginning to get used to this.

Avril rang, another of the women. She had heard me on the radio and saw me on the TV news the night before.

"Keep going. I wish I could do more," she said as she brought the radio to the phone so I could hear the local reaction coming in. It was more positive, a change from a year before.

"They come out of the woodwork when we talk about this," Paul said. He was fair-minded. I told Avril she gave me energy to keep going. We all had our different roles to play.

When I got to the Medical Council, I sat in reception waiting for Nicola, Cathriona, Jenny and Niamh as they sat upstairs, waiting one by one to give their evidence. My mobile rang. It was Christy Mannion, who worked in the Minister's office with Gobnait. "The Minister would like the women to come and see him on Tuesday the 24th at 11.00, if that is convenient."

I was very pleased, thinking we were getting somewhere after the news last night. The story of the opening of the hearing had been covered by RTÉ and TV3, and it even included an image of Neary arriving at the Council offices. I said I would pass on the message and get back to him. I could barely remember his name and of course I couldn't find a pen. I repeated Christy Mannion over and over, hoping that would make it stick. I left a message on Cathriona's mobile phone.

After this I needed a coffee. Only four women had told their stories the day before. The others were still waiting. And the wait was taking its toll on them all. They even talked about not being able to go through with their evidence, despite all their efforts.

Then Niamh came in with her mother. She was tired and grey. She had done it, told it as it was. They ordered coffee. Helen said, "She would win an Oscar for the way she hid her fear. She was so brave."

"Sure I heard Niamh tell her story the time we went to the Minister," I said. "Even the civil servants were crying. It's obvious she's telling the truth."

"My legs wouldn't stop shaking. I was trying to hide them so no one would see," Niamh said.

Her solicitor joined us then. "A stone would cry," she said. She looked flustered and, unusually for her, upset.

"You're upset too," I said.

She shook her head. She looked as if she were fighting back tears. Unsuccessfully.

Again the Neary entourage swept into the coffee shop. Niamh and the other women stiffened so much it was visible to everyone. A word from one of his company and Neary left as quickly as he had descended, without looking back.

We sat and talked. Niamh's mother again told us how she had persuaded Niamh to attend Neary. "I will not forgive myself," she said. Sorrow deepened and lowered Helen's voice as she spoke each word. In the end she was whispering.

"I should have known immediately," Niamh told us. "The social worker kept ringing me and asking if I needed any help after I came home."

The other women had joined us at the table by now. Niamh started to talk about the hearing. Through his barrister, Neary had denied everything. He still said he saved her life. "I was sitting at a table on my own, right in the middle of the room. A woman took me through the statement I made." This was the barrister, Mary Irvine.

"What was she like?"

"I felt she was on my side," was Niamh's reply. "Neary himself never spoke, though I kept catching his eye."

"Dear God, he has some nerve," Jenny referred to this and Neary's brief appearance and quick escape. She had spotted him returning to the Council offices.

"Maybe we should go back too in case they're looking for us," said Nicola. I stayed behind with Niamh and Helen.

That afternoon I sat and waited again in the Council's reception area. I was almost becoming a fixture there. Still, at least no one seemed to mind me. At the end of the second day, one of the women even told me where I could find coffee in Lynn House itself. While there I noticed the constant phone calls from doctors enquiring about registration, all of them with lovely foreign names, most of them polite when they were told registration only take calls between 2.45 and 4.00 p.m., but a large minority not very pleased at all. I wondered how they would deal with the cruelty and indignity of waiting to give evidence at a Medical Council inquiry. How would they deal with the secrecy? They called it confidentiality, but it was secrecy. And there was nowhere for patients to park here as they waited to tell their painful stories. The women had to keep dashing back and forth to buy a parking disc. I was amazed at how "patient" people were, at the level of discourtesy and pain they put up with to tell their stories. I am reminded of the philosopher, Nietzsche, who said, "He who has a why to live for can bear almost any how."

I saw fear too at the Medical Council during these days of waiting: a fear of the innocent, particularly those who have survived; a fear of the truth; a fear of ordinary language. The statutory body responsible for protecting the public was, it seemed, afraid of young women who have no wombs because of a bad doctor. They were afraid of me because I believed them. They presented secrecy as protection for the innocent, but it made the innocent ashamed. Shame and secrecy are bedfellows.

Could it be that the Medical Council felt responsible for the behaviour of Dr Neary – like a family where one member has gone bad? They shouldn't. Nothing is more liberating than being responsible only for your own behaviour. Good people became complicit not because they were guilty but because they were confused.

They were not gratuitously cruel in the Medical Council. They were just following the rules. I did not know then that some of them wanted to change these rules and were working towards it. Nor did I know then of the concerns some had for the integrity of the process, of their fear that we would derail their inquiry and so be instrumental in causing an application on Neary's behalf to the courts to have the inquiry ended.

The doctor, through his barrister, either denied everything or suggested that I was in some strange way responsible. The women told me that they were asked by the doctor's barrister if they were members of Patient Focus. I never heard of Neary before December 1998.

As I waited in reception, my mobile rang again. It was James, worrying about Nicola. "She is in telling her story right now," I told him. I knew this because Cathriona had phoned about two minutes earlier to see how I was. Tony arrived too. "She was coping fine at lunch. Nervous but fighting fit," I told James.

"Nicola puts on a great face, Sheila, but she's different inside," he said.

"I know. But the important thing is she can do it. She can put on that face." I had seen her eyes at lunch. The first time I ever noticed them and the clarity of purpose they held, as clear and sharp as blue African marble. "She will be fine," I said, because I have to say something to this man who will never have more children by the woman he so clearly loves and who loves him.

Then Jenny came in. It was over for her. She was the first of the women to go in after lunch. She was more relaxed than at lunch but she was still as if on a treadmill. She laughed and gave me a big hug.

"How was it?"

"Not too bad. He denied everything, of course. Didn't I know I might have a hysterectomy after my first baby? But I got an apology of sorts."

"What?" said Tony.

"Oh, the lady barrister said Dr Neary had no recollection of saying that he left the play pen and took away the cradle to you." Jenny mimicked the barrister's formality by changing her voice tone. "But if he did, he wishes me to say that it was never his intention to offend you in any way."

"She must have told him to give that apology anyway," Jenny said as she left to go back upstairs.

Tony was there so there was no need for me. "I'll head off home." As I got up to go, I noticed the portrait in reception of Dr Lynn, Ireland's first woman doctor. I wondered what she would think of this.

The rest of the women told their stories that afternoon. There was no need to go back to Lynn House again.

We went to see Micheál Martin on the Tuesday night. The meeting was moved back from 11.00 a.m. to 7.00 p.m.

"I can't go at that time," said Cathriona. "I'd have to come all the way back in from Kells. And I'm exhausted after the terrible time at the hearing. It's just not good enough. I've no time for him any more."

This delay embedded the growing distrust and turned it into a feeling that the women were wasting their time talking to the Minister for Health and Children.

Other women went, though, and told of their experiences with the Medical Council, the views of the English obstetrician and their frustration with the length of time everything took.

The Minister told us, "The Medical Council say that they will have completed hearings by February and I can't do anything till then."

Some weeks later a man rang to tell me of his own family's experience with Medical Council hearings. "They interrogated my wife. Wouldn't let me be with her as they questioned her. If we'd known this, our solicitor would have been there."

"We had a similar experience. It is uncivilised." I told him of the women leaving their husbands at home, of the right of the doctor in effect to decide who can be present at the hearing. My presence was vetoed.

"They wouldn't have told us of the result on our case if we had not been there at the time. You mightn't be told the result."

"Thanks for that warning. We'll try and look out for that."

"How can you talk openly about it? What about their confidentiality?" he asked, sounding confused.

"This is a democratic country," I replied. "We have a written constitution. We are only talking about the fact that the hearing is happening. So far no one has written to me to tell me I have broken some law. Anyway, it's different for me. I'm not fighting my own fight so I'm not nervous. I think they have far more to fear from the truth than me."

"I've been there. I understand. I also know this must stop. Good caring people traumatised by medical treatment," he said, after about half an hour on the phone. "My solicitor says it's a public duty to tell the truth about what happened to us."

"Would you like to help us put in place suggestions as to how the Medical Council needs to be improved?"

"I'd love to," he said. "The whole system needs to be changed."

"Questioning the way things are done will improve the practice of medicine far more than pumping another billion pounds into it."

"There's nothing surer," he said.

I wished him and his family luck in their struggle and said I would be in touch. No more silence. No more lives destroyed by it. That was his message to us.

In Lynn House they had to be made to understand this: that sometimes people need protection from doctoring.

7

Mixed Messages

In December 2000 a letter from Margaret Carroll, the convenor of the Curriculum Development Committee, gave me my opportunity to advance the communication process between the Lourdes maternity unit and the women. Topics for the agenda of the next meeting were being invited. I emailed my proposal that representatives of women I work with be invited to tell the Committee of their experiences and later to speak to the students themselves.

On the night before the meeting, Margaret rang with a problem. "The problem with women from your group talking to the committee is that a woman might be talking to a committee member who looked after her when she was having her baby."

I hadn't expected this reason. I suggested leaving it off the agenda for the following day's meeting and that we make an arrangement for her, Tony and I to discuss it after Christmas.

"Okay," she said. "Some Wednesday in January."

I felt I had got somewhere. Beginning to make an omelette without breaking too many eggs.

Just before the following morning's meeting, another member of the committee came up to me. "Are you Sheila?" She stretched out her hand in greeting. "I'm Mary, a midwifery advisor from Holles Street."

"I'm here because I accidentally became involved in a support group of women badly damaged in Drogheda," I said.

"I know. I've seen the results of Neary's work in Holles Street." She was referring to women who attended there for remedial medical care as a result of Neary's work. *Keep it up*, was Mary's unspoken message. Maybe I was not as much an outsider as I thought.

Some days later, Linda, one of the women, rang to say her letter asking for others who may have been damaged in the Lourdes Hospital to get in touch was published in the *Drogheda Independent*. Later that evening, she rang again. She had got an abusive call.

"What about the people in the hospital? They're being witch-hunted. What about the nurses, the consultants?" the anonymous woman had said.

"You couldn't reason with her. She just wanted to give out," Linda explained.

"Ask the editor to give my number or Tony's in future."

"I'll give it another shot," Linda said. She believed there were a lot more women out there like her. They would benefit from the group. The women were really wonderful, I thought.

As I was musing on this I opened my email. It was from my daughter Aideen. It contained a photo from an article called "The Rescuing Hug". The article told the story of newborn twin girls. They were in separate incubators. One was not expected to live. A hospital nurse fought against the rules and put them together in one incubator. The healthier of the twins put an arm over her sister in a sweet hug. The smaller baby's heart rate stabilised, her temperature rose to normal and she survived. I loved it. The twins, bare except for nappies, faces towards each other, were smaller, much smaller than their nappies. To me they embody what it is to be human. They are all of us at some time. And we will need that nurse. We would keep going and recruit the nurses somehow.

Tony and I met Margaret from the Curriculum Development Committee on a cold crisp day in January. At the start she told us a little about herself. She had long experience at home and abroad as a midwife and teacher. She was clearly the lynchpin of this important pilot course.

I suggested introducing a module into the programme whereby midwives were encouraged to be brave, to speak up when things were wrong, starting off with minor matters and working up to more serious. Teaching people how to react before they actually find themselves in difficult situations. Trial runs, like fire drill.

"You must teach people to come between doctors and patients when it is needed," Tony said. Margaret agreed. "You can teach anyone to be a good communicator," Tony said. He was framing the suggestion as a communication module in the curriculum.

"What if one of the women who came to talk to the students was looked after by one of our midwives?" she asked.

"That can happen in the town," Tony said. "In shops, on the street. They can meet anywhere."

"But it would affect the relationship between the student and her teacher," she said.

"It probably does anyway. There has been lots of publicity in the press. It must have been seen. It can only increase. The women want an independent, public inquiry. The Neary story will be before the High Court by the end of the year, as a number of cases are in preparation and one or two are likely to come to court soon," I said.

"What happened in the Lourdes anyway?" Margaret asked. She didn't know! She had been away, and no one had told her. She was on a committee with many women who worked in the maternity unit of the Lourdes, and no one had told her. I had assumed she knew. Tony and I told her briefly of Neary's unnecessary surgery. She visibly winced and looked upset.

Tony and I suggested talking just to the committee as a compromise. "You will see how forgiving patients can be," he said, "how they are quite sane even after what happened them."

"And in this case," I said, "it was midwives who blew the whistle. Don't forget that. We need to celebrate that."

Margaret still seemed concerned.

Still trying, I said, "I understand many of the midwives went home crying in the evening for a while before the plug was pulled on the obstetrician. People feel terrible when these things are happening – much worse than they do when they do the proper thing."

Margaret still had concerns, and the meeting ended with no firm commitments.

Noreen's Story

Noreen comes from the Georgian village of Slane. It is not just famous for its castle and rock concerts; close by is the Hill of Slane, where it is said the first Easter fire was lit by St Patrick to symbolise the arrival of Christianity to Ireland. The act was in direct defiance of the Celtic King of Ireland. Noreen must have been imbued with that sense of defiance as she tried to mend her broken heart after the hurt Neary caused her. This warm and spunky lady was in her late forties at the time of her gynaecological surgery.

"It was a vaginal hysterectomy that went wrong," she told me. Its consequences destroyed her life. When she awoke after her operation, Neary told her he couldn't do the hysterectomy because "the time ran out". She was in terrible pain following this surgery.

A few months later, he rearranged the hysterectomy and this time removed her ovaries as well. But the pain still remained. It was so bad, Noreen couldn't sit down. The extreme pain prevented her from sharing a bed with her husband and she was forever unable to have a full sexual relationship with him. She was also incontinent. This distressed them both terribly.

Eventually, she sought a second opinion in a Dublin hospital. Reconstructive surgery was arranged and this made an enormous difference to her. At this clinic, she was told the surgery left her destroyed internally. "You wouldn't see it in the backstreets of Calcutta," she was told.

"I had to sleep on my own after Neary," she told me. "I needed the whole bed to be able to drop off. The terrible pain is gone and I am not incontinent, but Neary destroyed my life. Only that I had a wonderful husband he would have ruined my marriage too. After him, we could only kiss. He sewed me up so tight. The truth about what he did must come out. My husband died recently and the loneliness is terrible. I want this to come out for him. Please put it in a book. I want to see it in a book. My husband was a good man who loved me and I couldn't love him back in his last few years."

Noreen's story is representative of several mature women who suffered in this way as a result of Neary's gynaecological techniques. Dr Neary was not found guilty in her case at the Medical Council.

8

A Politician is Interested

Everyone was tired in January 2000, especially the women who had been to the Medical Council. Cross-examination by a barrister can fragment you. The women had read medical reports of the negligent care they received, they had told their stories to solicitors and read their statements back, but defending it to a "court" makes it even more real. The spoken word is more immediate, more in your face, and defending it requires access to your soul. Many of the women were feeling sort of broken. Christmas is always a bad time, but this year it seemed especially terrible.

I thought about what the women said about Neary. About how he appeared to go on binges of unnecessary surgery. They knew of two occasions where he performed two caesarean hysterectomies in one night. How January seemed to be a bad month for them. About how the numbers in our group were still growing – about sixty in all now, and most were taking legal action. Three out of four cases referred by solicitors for medico-legal opinions came back with the opinion that their surgery was unnecessary. I thought about how Neary seemed to be getting worse as the years went on, about how charming he was to some women and very abusive to others, how difficult it was to bring it all to public attention. It was very hard on the women to do this job. Everything took so long, the women thought it a form of institutional abuse. They wanted to work for change.

These thoughts were interrupted by a ringing phone.

"Could I speak to Sheila O Connor?" a woman's voice said. I didn't recognise it so I thought it might be a new woman.

"Speaking."

"This is Liz McManus. I'm Labour spokesperson for Health," she said. "I got your number from Ruairi Quinn, the Labour Party leader. You rang his office."

"That's ages ago, well before Christmas."

"Sorry it took so long to get back to you."

"Oh no, no," I said. "We were all very tired before Christmas anyway. I would have got on to you soon anyway. You know what it is in relation to?"

"The Drogheda obstetrician. I have referred to it in public before," she said.

"You couldn't really know about it unless you knew people closely involved. It's a terrible story." I filled her in on the details – the number of women involved; length of time; difficulties with the Medical Council; the situation with Micheál Martin, how difficult it was to be cross with him. He looked so worried.

I told her we wanted a public independent inquiry. I referred to the people who let this go on for so long and told her details of the medico-legal reports coming back – no blood necessary, normal wombs, etc. She invited us to come and see her in the Dáil and invited us to lunch in the Dáil restaurant.

"I'll bring some of the women with me," I said.

Liz McManus sounded shocked at the story.

"The Medical Council should be there to protect patients, not doctors," she said. "There is no reason why there should not be a public inquiry; the sooner the better. The Medical Council does its own business, the Minister should do his. This is a matter of public importance. This should be investigated. It demonstrates the same mindset as the babies' organs scandal. You couldn't get anything more perfect to push for change."

"The women in our group are the people to do it. They are becoming so empowered; it is so good to see it. Wait till you meet them," I said.

"That's great, I look forward to that." She meant it. So did I.

Setting up the visit to Liz McManus was easy.

"It is now almost becoming routine, going to Dublin," Nicola said when I rang her.

"I know, it's the same for me. Amazing, isn't it?" I replied.

"In the beginning I used to shake but now it's just another visit to the Dáil to meet a politician," she laughed. Nicola always laughs. But this time it was deep. She was amused at herself.

"I'm sure I can go. What's the date?"

"The 24th. You've plenty time to think about it. If you can't, I have time to get someone else, so don't feel you have to. No need for personal stories any more, unless you want to," I said.

"My sister says, why am I putting it on myself," Nicola continues, "but I think it normal now."

"Even after the Medical Council?" I ask.

"After that, I can do anything."

Clearly I was worrying too much. Nicola was one strong lady. "I think so, too. You'll never look back really now, Nicola."

I know in my soul that is true. Nicola is a new woman.

Niamh, Noreen, Cathriona and Jenny are just as easy to persuade. They all jump at the suggestion. This will be Noreen's first visit. But she is all set immediately. She has been in the group since the early days.

"I still cry nearly every night," she says. "You know I'm game. We have to do this."

I know and we do indeed. Noreen is very gutsy. The type of woman who would never let anyone down. She needed no more than to be asked and she was off to do what should be done.

"Liz McManus has asked us to lunch in the Dáil afterwards. I think that's the least you deserve," I said to Noreen.

"So do I."

"I'm serious," I said, unsure of her tone.

"So am I," she said in a tone which said she was never more sure of anything.

Cathriona took a day off work, even though she had just started a new job.

Niamh said Sean, her partner, might come this time if he can get the time off.

"Great," I said. "That would be great."

I arrived first at Buswell's. Noreen arrived moments later.

"Well, there's me and you anyway," she said in her own resigned way. Nicola arrived soon after, casually dressed in a body warmer and jeans. I took this as proof that she was feeling more at ease; dressed for travel and action.

"Oh, the others will be here very soon, don't worry." Cathriona and Jenny were in view.

"I wonder how many more times will we meet like this?" Jenny asked.

"As many as it takes," said Cathriona. She meant it.

Niamh arrived with Sean. A lovely fair-haired young man, no more than twenty-three or so, the same as my son Dave. I shook hands as I was introduced to this tall, quiet-spoken young man who wore glasses. I thought of him being kept out of the delivery room as his partner, the mother of his baby, had her womb removed. I stopped my mind racing. It was time to go to meet Liz McManus.

This meeting was in the new building, Leinster House 2000. To get there you pass through a glass foyer; very twenty-first century. The meeting room had a large oval table in the centre. We sat ourselves down on either side. After a few moments Liz McManus came in and sat at the top of the table.

She was dressed in black, her long slim skirt and neat-fitting little top set off with a silver scarf and jumbo pearls. She introduced herself. I introduced everyone to her. Cathriona, Jenny, Sean and Niamh, Nicola and Noreen. Liz McManus welcomed us, told us this was our place. We were at home here.

"That's as it should be in a democracy," she said. She told us she had just been at a meeting of the Joint Oireachtas Committee of Health and Children (JOCHC) and our recent letter requesting them to hear the women's stories was read out. The Minister told the committee the matter was with the Medical Council. The committee would get back to us.

Cathriona handed her the dossier of questionnaires filled in by many of the women, their personal testimonies. Everyone spoke about their personal experiences at the hospital. They told of how they had just been witnesses at the Medical Council, how they had been made to feel as if it was none of their business, how they had waited around for two days to give their evidence, the secrecy surrounding the venue.

"Everyone was very upset after the Medical Council," Cathriona said. "It was very hard. This is so personal to every woman and he was there looking at you."

"And they don't even have to tell you what they decide," someone else chimed in.

Liz listened. "I didn't fully realise the seriousness of this issue before," she said when it was all told. Niamh cried a little. Sean comforted her. No one was embarrassed except Niamh. We explained that we wanted the Labour Party to support an investigation into the hospital and the eventual establishment of a compensation tribunal. Liz nodded and agreed. We expected an election soon and wanted Labour to have this as part of any election manifesto. She nodded again.

It was time for lunch in the Dáil restaurant, which is like a small hotel dining room, intimate yet formal. Each circular table is covered in a white tablecloth, a flower arrangement in the centre, lots of cutlery carefully positioned, linen serviettes, wine glasses, menus, a feeling of clutter and etiquette. It's old-fashioned and comfortable. I got the feeling of being at home, but still it was a treat. Our table was all ready for us, set for eight. I spot prominent politicians everywhere – Alan Dukes, Mary Harney, Liz O'Donnell, Alan Shatter at a table by himself. No sooner are we seated than Des Hanafin stops to chat to Liz. He is on his way out. She introduces us as a group of ladies from Drogheda.

By the time we finished our meal and got to the coffee, there were very few left in the restaurant.

"You have to keep at it," Liz McManus said. "I will raise it in the Dáil, get others to do it too, keep it in front of the civil servants and the Minister."

"We'll pester them all right," Cathriona said. "Nothing surer."

We all agreed we were only beginning.

On the way out, the front of Leinster House was crawling with journalists. Ursula Halligan, a journalist with TV3, was in the centre of the plinth.

"Do you think they're waiting for us," quipped Jenny, "or do you think its Liam Lawlor they're after?"

"It's probably Liam today but one day it will be us," Cathriona said.

The phone rang again at lunchtime on 28 February. It was Liz McManus again.

"I put down a parliamentary question about the Neary issue. It's for answer this afternoon. Could you come? It's for oral reply, to be taken at about 3.15 or so."

"Yes, I'll go in. I'd make it if I left now and parked in Setanta. I've enough time for that."

"Could I just check something with you – he was doing caesarean hysterectomies for about twenty-one years; is that right?"

"Probably longer than that. The oldest baby in our group is twenty-one, if you know what I mean, but not everyone is in our group."

"Thanks. I'll leave a message at security so you can get in."

"Thank you, Liz," my voice was rising.

Aideen of course isn't in from school yet. Katie is here though so she agrees to check on her. Just then the door bell rings. Luckily for once it's Aideen.

"I'm going in to the Dáil," I say. "Would anyone like to come with me?"

"I've to do an essay," said Katie.

"No, I don't think so," Aideen said. "Do you want to try my soup?" She pointed to a tub of soup she had made in school.

"No time," I said, grabbing a bag of crisps and a bar of chocolate and checking I had money for parking. Off I went into the cold. It had been snowing.

The Dáil is not that impressive. Once inside, I am afraid to make a noise. Its circular chamber is decorated with gold curtains to the back and a royal blue carpet with a gold Celtic pattern. All the seats are in brown leather. Most were empty when I got there. I ate my Turkish Delight and nobody said anything so that must be allowed. I moved to a better seat where I would be able to see the Minister when he spoke.

I recalled the last time I had been there. It was the night of the debate about the women who had contracted hepatitis C from contaminated blood they received from the Irish Blood Transfusion Service. The night Michael Noonan, who was Minister for Health at the time, said that the legal advisors to Brigid McCole, one of the infected women who was seriously ill, would be better advised picking the case of a woman who was in better condition. The Positive Action women had walked out of the Dáil in disgust. He was there again today, questioning the Taoiseach on Sinn Féin this time. He was very polite, amazingly polished.

At about 3.25, it was the turn of questions to Micheál Martin and Mary Hanafin. Ironically, the first question related to the adoption of foreign children by childless Irish couples and what Gay Mitchell called unnecessary bureaucratic delays. Then it was the turn of the question I had come to hear. It was not read out; each question had a number. The Minister proceeded to his answer. Nobody in the public gallery could know the question.

He emphasised that it was a very sensitive issue which had been adequately dealt with by the NEHB once it was brought to their attention. He outlined the findings of the IOG's review. He talked of the ongoing Medical Council hearings. He told of his meetings with Patient Focus and of how he went to Drogheda and met the women and their families. He would await the Medical Council decision before deciding on any action. He added that he was not ruling anything out.

Liz McManus rose to ask a supplementary question. "I understand this is very sensitive question. But it is very serious and relates to what can only be described as the systematic, unnecessary mutilation of women of child-bearing age, maybe as many as ninety women over twenty-one years. In the end it became almost a daily occurrence. Is the Minister not aware that, despite the Health Board actions and the Medical Council, which is only considering one individual, many others must have been involved in this practice and yet nobody blew the whistle until two young nurses could take it no longer? It is the Minister's duty to find out the truth and to ensure it never happens again. Is the Minister aware that consultants can become mentally ill or do wrong in other ways and it will no longer do to leave everything to them?"

"Will the deputy stick to the question?" said the Ceann Comhairle.

The Minister responded, "I don't want to prejudge the content of that inquiry or make remarks that might appear to prejudge it. I formed a judgement . . . it seemed logical to await the . . . Medical Council." He added that the Medical Council was telling him that it would reach its decision by February, but obviously he couldn't interfere with them. He did however say he was ruling nothing out. He emphasised that and, of course, he wanted to find out the truth. And it was a hospital matter and not just one individual, he said.

By that stage I had stopped taking notes because a lovely usher told me gently, even with a hint of embarrassment in his voice and a "sorry about that" look on his face, that I shouldn't take notes in there. I stopped in case I got this lovely man and myself into trouble.

I was happy. At least here the truth was spoken, even if to very few people.

I would tell everyone tomorrow. No one mentioned that this was the last day of February and that the date now being floated by the Medical Council for a decision was autumn. But I still thought we were getting places and that day I celebrated a country where, now at least, things were starting to come out. Or maybe it was just the surroundings, the impressive trappings of democracy where the citizen was definitely welcome and Deputy Liz McManus spoke the truth.

I rang Jenny to tell her. She had been very down. I read my notes over to her.

"It's the truth," she said. "It's terrible that the Medical Council hearing is taking so long. They don't take our feelings into account. We are really locked out; you were locked out. And it is all about us. I don't want Neary calling himself 'doctor'. That is what it means to me. His healer's title needs to be gone."

Next morning I rang Liz's office to thank her for the speech. I asked to speak to her. Her assistant seemed reticent when I said it was in connection with the Drogheda hospital scandal and her speech in the Dáil. I explained myself a little more. I wanted to thank her for being so forthright. For saying it like it was. I wanted to tell her of the reaction of the women.

She lightened up. "Liz has been getting phone calls here from people saying they will do everything they can from now on to ruin her life because of what she said in the Dáil about the hospital and the doctor. We do everything we can to protect Liz from this sort of thing."

"Of course," I said. "That's terrible. Well then, just tell her I called."

"People like Neary always have supporters," she said.

"As far as I am concerned, they're like groupies," I said.

I remembered the threatening phone call Linda got when she wrote a letter to the local paper asking if there were any others who wished to join our group. It was from someone who said they worked in the hospital. Linda hadn't been in touch since. It frightened her. What was these people's problem?

The following Monday I got a rather confused letter. The writer was organising a petition to the Minister for Health complaining about Patient Focus and Liz McManus. The writer claimed to have received "several thousand" phone calls of complaint about us and Liz.

9

Straight Talk

The snow was hard and crisp after the previous night's frost as I headed off to meet the women and the Tánaiste, Mary Harney. We were to meet her at noon in her office. The traffic was light so I got in easily to our Buswell's Hotel rendezvous. We were almost regulars there now. Noreen was standing at the hotel door. She looked upset, I realised, as I got nearer. She spotted me.

"I thought no one was coming. I'm the only one here."

We are all very fond of Noreen. A good person, a woman with real guts, and heart. She struggled on her own for years to show how she had been mutilated by Neary, but got nowhere. She was helped and improved by another obstetrician. However, she had no written report to prove how badly Neary damaged her. A piece of her file was missing and a later excellent doctor treated her and improved her condition very much, leaving insufficient evidence of Neary's work. She was told she would get used to it: to having no relationship with her beloved husband, to the scars, to the pain.

"It looks horrible. Isn't it terrible to say that?" she said once to me.

There was pain in her face as she stood in the cold at the door of Buswell's. She had left home at 7.30 to get there on the bus. Mary Harney's secretary had put back the meeting from 11.30 to noon, but I never told Noreen of the delay because I expected everyone to be early. She was just about to go off to phone. I apologised and felt terrible, but Noreen said never mind, shrugged it off.

We waited in the hotel foyer for the others. I told Noreen about Liz McManus and her plain language in the Dáil, about her use of the word "mutilation".

"It's the truth," she says, determination in her voice. "The Dáil is the only place where you can speak the truth in Ireland now, about Neary and Drogheda anyway. Even *The Irish Times* avoids mention of this issue. The paper that broke the story. Today there is no mention of Liz's Dáil question in its Dáil Report."

Tony, Maura and her husband Pat arrive. Maura suffered severe gynaecological damage and wanted to do something to prevent this happening to others. "No nerves today," she said. "And we are going to see the second most powerful person in the country. We must be getting places."

Maura took a letter from her pocket signed by Micheál Martin to a local TD. It was the first written acknowledgement we got that he was asked for an inquiry. Yesterday in the Dáil was the first public, verbal one. We were beginning to feel that from little acorns great oaks grow.

Nicola rang. She was coming after all. She was on the train but would be a little late. We headed across to the Dáil. We announced ourselves to security and waited in their Kildare Street hut. The Tánaiste was not in her office, we were told.

Nicola rang again, still on the train. We were to go on without her. She would join us soon. I sorted matters with security men so she could join us.

By that stage Mary Harney's assistant had arrived. She didn't know what was happening; the Tánaiste was in the Dáil.

"This is very important and people here have come a long way," I said.

She was upset. "It's nothing to do with me; I can't help it. I know nothing about this."

I felt bad, thinking I had harassed her. Maybe I had. She made a phone call; no luck, no answer. We persisted. She left, very upset. We stayed. And waited. Nicola arrived. Catherine Bulbulia, the Tánaiste's advisor, arrived too and took over, calm and in control. We discovered we were in the wrong place. We had to meet Mary Harney in her Department office, not her Dáil one. Catherine would show us over. A crisis meeting about foot and mouth was taking place and the Tánaiste had to attend. But she would meet us, we were reassured.

We crossed the road to the Department of Enterprise, Trade and Employment, and were taken to a waiting area on the first floor. We were met there by John O'Brien, one of the Tánaiste's team.

"We will get things under way ourselves. The Tánaiste will join us as soon as she can. But she *will* join us," he emphasised. He must have sensed scepticism.

The Tánaiste's room had a swing leather chair behind a wooden desk, much as I remembered a principal officer's office from my time in the civil service. There was a circular table in the corner with eight or ten chairs around it. It was a small enough room. The only difference was that Mary Harney had an inner office and her staff were in another room outside.

Maura started the meeting, introduced everyone and summarised the problem. She had set it up originally by writing to the Tánaiste. We were also keen to meet her as leader of the Progressive Democrats party. They did not have a Dáil member in the Louth Meath area.

Maura was composed and articulate, no sign of the shake that was in my voice when I did this job at our first meeting with Micheál Martin. Just then Mary Harney arrived, took a seat at the table and got down to business. No introductions here, no small talk. Her body language seemed to say: let's hear the facts, tell me what you want and how you think I can help. Maura told her of Liz McManus and of Micheál Martin's response. I said I felt like crying in the Dáil the day before listening to Liz's straight talk. We tried to fill her in on as much of the detail as we could, as quickly as possible. She apologised for the mix-up in location and time and referred to the foot-and-mouth crisis. But she listened. Tony spoke of the Medical Council and how no one knew when it was going to reach a decision. Everyone said something except Pat. As ever, the men were supportive but did not intrude.

"The main point," the Tánaiste said, "is that the Medical Council and the hospital issue are separate and need not be linked to one another." She added, "So you want an inquiry?"

She took out Maura's handwritten letter seeking to meet her and read it. Tony said he felt Micheál Martin would like to announce an inquiry but maybe needed a nudge along.

"I understand. I support you in this." She was clear, no fuss, no sweet talk, no bonding. Just clear.

The Tánaiste rose. She had to go. "The Taoiseach is away today and there is this crisis. I am pleased to have met you and I will talk to Micheál Martin and get back to you. In about two weeks or so." She left quietly.

As we gathered our things I said to John O'Brien, "I don't know why I think of Neary together with the other consultant in that hospital who is up before the courts accused of indecently assaulting young boys over a thirty-year period. It must be because he and Neary were friends."

The following Monday I got a letter from Maura, enclosing a copy of the report of Liz McManus's Dáil speech in the *Irish Independent* of Thursday, 1 March. It was headed "WOMEN MUTILATED IN HOSPITAL". I could see why it upset people. The truth tends to when starkly put.

Later in March it hit me why what transpired in the Dáil between Micheál Martin and Liz McManus was so important. At last clear language had been used in public by a public representative. It made the truth much easier to accept.

Our next trip to Leinster House was on 28 March, to see Michael Noonan. He had recently been elected leader of Fine Gael. Maura again set up the meeting. For most of March I mulled over Neary and his activities like a cow chews the cud, as my dad would have said. Not in a depressive way. Tony and I were discussing it too. Liz

McManus's language in the Dáil seemed to release restrictions, as did the fact that some papers published it. At least, the *Irish Independent* did. The insights that came to me, though brutal, were a relief.

The meeting with the politicians was in the Leinster House Millennium Building again. The meeting was prompt and we were shown by a lovely, friendly, funny woman to Michael Noonan's office. We joked that we had nothing to wear for political action of a lobbying kind now instead of talking about how nervous we were.

"I have plenty of clothes for washing up, collecting kids from school, even a few glamorous silk and velvet things, but nothing for this," said Maura. She is always very smart, I thought.

In the end I wore my big fluffy jumper with a chiffon scarf and black trousers. I had spent ages looking for it. I eased the creases from it, polished my shoes and I was ready to go. Maura, her husband Pat and Rosemary Cunningham, who also complained to the Medical Council about her treatment by Neary, were waiting, though I was early.

Michael Noonan stood up as we entered and we all introduced ourselves. Within a few minutes Gay Mitchell joined the meeting. The office was modern and new, with the ubiquitous round table. Michael Noonan seemed shy to start the conversation. We chatted about topical issues for a few minutes first. Then both Rosemary and Maura told their stories of the serious gynaecological damage they experienced at the hands of Neary. I filled in the generalities.

This meeting was more informal and more honest than the others. Gone was the concern about making a presentation, about appearing ultra-reasonable. The tone was quiet and restrained though the content was open and frank. But terrible things were said.

"There are inefficient doctors and even bad doctors, as we have seen from the tribunals. But this is different," we said. Gay Mitchell asked about Neary's wife and her death. He had heard that the reason Neary was so out of order was because of upset at his wife's death from ovarian cancer. But his wife died in 1996. We told these two men the whole story again.

It was interesting how we were comforting these men in their embarrassment. Much like people don't know what to say at a wake. Neither man seemed to know what to say. Maybe we were blasting them with information.

Michael asked if Neary acknowledged responsibility and we said no, he was refusing to accept anything. Then we said that doctors can be mentally ill or personality-disordered too. I commented how he appeared to want to strip women of everything female.

Other issues in the hospital were commented on – that is, how another senior doctor in the hospital was facing charges of sexual assault on several teenage boys and that these two men were friends.

People believe it when a doctor tells them he saved their life, we said. They want to, even need to. Like children believe their mothers when she says she loves them. Otherwise they are faced with a very special betrayal.

Both men nodded and agreed. Gay Mitchell promised to raise a parliamentary question in the Dáil regarding the length of time the Minister for Health was willing to await an adjudication from the Medical Council. We discussed the Oireachtas Committee on Health and Children. Michael

Noonan kept commenting how it was shocking. We told them we wanted to be able to say when this was all over that the NEHB did well and so did the politicians.

In the end I asked if they believed us. They said, "of course." Gay Mitchell's eyes suggested he did. I couldn't see Michael Noonan's as I sat beside him but his body language was very reassuring. Gay Mitchell referred to Fine Gael's policy of a health ombudsman in their latest manifesto and the need to revise the Medical Practitioners Act.

We all agreed this was necessary.

The informality of it was good. How we had grown. And we would get there in the end with the help of good people. That is what it was all about. That is how one recovers. There must be no unreachables any more and no disposable people either. Everyone was answerable. Healing must come from this.

Our meeting was both frank and subdued at the same time, like a wake.

On Friday 30 March I phoned Gay Mitchell and left a message of thanks on his answering machine for their time and attention. I specifically made the point that we in Patient Focus were not in the business of blaming politicians for what doctors had done. I added that I believed that Michael Noonan in particular got a lot of stick over the hepatitis C case. So much so, one would be forgiven for thinking that he had personally poisoned the blood himself.

10

An Oireachtas Committee

In early May I attended a meeting of the Health Strategy Forum. Tony and I tried to use every opportunity to bring the women's experience to "health service stakeholders". This was our opportunity to influence the content of a new health strategy regarding the need for patient advocacy. My stomach was growing increasingly delicate at that time. I could not cope with what I knew went on in the Lourdes.

It is important to be angry because people who are badly treated either blame themselves for what happened to them or scrounge around with the air of a small-time thief looking for someone somewhere to help them. They are more likely to be refused help on the grounds that they are imagining things than they are to be helped. That is the reality. That is why patient advocacy was important and must be a real part of this new health strategy. The need for a wide investigation into Drogheda was writ large in my brain too; otherwise people would never believe. It would happen again. To ensure it doesn't happen again, an advocacy service is needed for patients.

"Medical professionals don't like the expression 'patient advocacy'," I was told at the small group session on quality at the forum when I said that advocacy matters. I couldn't believe it. "They are threatened by advocacy," the group session participant added.

"They don't like the word 'complaint' either," another participant said. Why don't they like these plain words? What is wrong with these words?

As I was reflecting on this discussion, and feeling totally fed up, the phone rang. It was John Hamilton from the Joint Oireachtas Committee on Health and Children inviting Patient Focus to make a presentation to a full meeting of the committee on Thursday 10 May. It had a two-hour slot. We would speak at 9.45 with questions and answers after that. We wrote to the committee chairman, Batt O'Keeffe, asking that they set up an inquiry. The Green Party's health spokesperson, John Gormley, had suggested this as a possible alternative route to obtaining an inquiry. We had met John Gormley the previous December. He was helpful and the women said they got good vibes from him. Niamh, Majella and Jack, Maura and Pat, and Iseult, were all at the meeting. He assured us the Greens would support any moves to institute an inquiry. They would even have it high on their "shopping list" if they were power-brokers following the election we all expected in summer 2002.

I rang John Hamilton back later to ask him about privilege before the committee.

"It has never been tested," he said, "but the committee's legal advice is that witnesses have qualified privilege. The same as when giving evidence before the High Court. Members have absolute privilege but witnesses have qualified privilege." As a careful addition, he emphasised: "But I cannot guarantee that."

Nicola agreed to come as the women's representative. After our experience in Lynn House, I checked with the committee that we would all be let in together. We would.

"What would your Dad think of you doing this?" I asked her.

"He'd be delighted. He was a great man himself for going to TDs." Nicola was laughing. She always spoke very fondly of her dad, of how he encouraged her to engage in life again. I imagined him with a cap on, banging on doors to ensure they opened, not going until he got satisfaction about whatever was up. I imagined him as an honourable countryman, someone who knew right from wrong. I imagined him with a broken heart over his beautiful and equally honourable daughter. She was now fighting the honourable fight with the bravery of a lion and the kindness of a lovebird.

"I think he even took it worse than my mother," Nicola said. "He bottled everything up; he never talked about it much."

I spent the next few days preparing the submission. I checked a few details, counted out my list of names, the sixty-five or so taking legal action, the number who had caesarean hysterectomies, the numbers who were Neary patients, the small numbers who were patients of other doctors, the number of gynaecology patients. I spoke with our legal advisor, Colm MacGeehin.

"Drogheda deserves an investigation of its own," he said. "It was a terrible place. An inquiry and a compensation tribunal are necessary. One like the Stardust, one that gives proper compensation, commensurate with damage. And some women are not able to go to court. They haven't even told their mothers. And then there's the missing files. Of course, from a legal perspective of the hospital or doctor, the best defence is missing or destroyed files."

Colm and Tony strengthened my initial draft. Colm said I should include the word "dishonestly" in relation to Neary telling women he saved their lives. We should also say "the removal of wombs without consent amounted to serious criminal assault".

"Can I say that?"

"Of course you can. It's in private. You have qualified privilege. That means you can say anything so long as it is not with malice and it is true to your knowledge."

"Yes," I thought, "I have a duty to tell what I believe happened."

Next morning I emailed the submission to John Hamilton and to Tony. Then the phone rang.

"It's bad news," said Nicola. "I can't go to the committee. James is needed at the Medical Council. He has to tell them who he talked to after my operation." So the hearings were still going on? We were unaware of what stage had been reached or how much longer it would take.

"That's okay, Nicola. I'm delighted for James. He will get his say at last. Neary will be sorry he made James come in. Wait till the Council hear his story. If I was Neary's lawyer I wouldn't let him talk, that's for sure. I'll find someone else. Don't worry."

"James has to identify Neary. He is denying he did the operation. He signed nothing, you see. He says it was another doctor who did it." Nicola reminded me that she'd had a general anaesthetic, unlike the later women, who had epidurals, so she doesn't remember.

"God knows what he did to me when I was asleep. I won't go there anyway."

"No."

"I hope James will keep his cool."

"Oh, of course he will," I said.

"He's really mad. I can't guarantee what he will do when he sees 'that man' as he calls him."

"Tell him I said not to hit him."

"He says he can't guarantee that."

"Okay, tell him not to hit him tomorrow. Not at the Medical Council anyway, not in Portobello. Some other time. Take it one day at a time. Just promise not to do it tomorrow," I said. We were both laughing by this stage, knowing James would never do such a thing. "Good luck. Give me a ring and let me know how it goes. If he needs me to go down I will."

I needed to find another woman at very short notice. But Tony said we could represent them well by then. He was looking forward to it. I was reassured, just for a while. But who was I to talk for the women? This doubt lingered and grew. I still had to do it, though. It was too late.

I met Tony at 9.15 after an Aideen morning.

"Will you hurry up," I said. "I'll be late." She was still walking round half asleep at 7.50 and we had to leave at 8.00 and have breakfast as well. Her friend Catherine too. She had stayed overnight. She was even less ready.

"Breakfast's in the car; that's all that's for it." They both climbed in, still getting dressed, still eating breakfast, still combing hair.

"Teenagers are a big pain," I tell them that too.

"See my new tie," Aideen said, changing the subject as she tied it around her neck – loose, you understand; can't have it neat up at the neck.

"Where did you get that?"

"Catherine stole it for me from lost property."

"Did she now?" I was unsure about how to handle this. She was someone else's child. She was in the car listening. Discretion is the better part of valour, I decided. I didn't say anything about anything.

The table in the committee room was a polished circle with chairs all around – about twenty-five in all. The chairman with his secretariat sat at the top, while two people sat in a recess in the wall, whom I assumed were recording proceedings. This time the JOCHC was sitting in private session.

Tony and I sat down at the place marked for us. After initial introductions I explained Nicola's absence, emphasising the short notice from the Medical Council. I started off but was very nervous, so I handed over to Tony to explain what a caesarean hysterectomy is. I regained my breath and helped myself to some water. Then I explained the history, as I had done so many times before, but this time in greater detail. I explained the tragedy of the hospital and what they had done. Everyone listened. I mentioned Nicola's story again of how she was expecting to be discharged when Neary, who was not even her doctor, decided she needed a section, then a hysterectomy – none of it necessary, according to Irish and British medico-legal reports.

"Neary may have been a monster who damaged women. This is a possibility we need to bear in mind," Tony said at the close of the presentation.

I couldn't judge how we were received. I was on automatic pilot. Tony said it was fine. So did Liz McManus, who came over to introduce herself to Tony.

I rang Nicola when I got home. There were messages from the women wishing me luck. A friend made me tea. I relaxed for the first time in ages as I talked to her and told her I hoped we did well, but I didn't know.

Next morning I talked to Sandra, whose baby had died. She had medical reports saying it shouldn't have happened. She was grieving for her precious lost baby. Sandra had had another baby since, who was two months old at that time. But she still missed her little child. I told her I had informed the committee of the two dead babies in writing.

"But why don't they listen to women, to what they tell them? I think that is what happened to my baby. Nobody listened to me. I kept telling them but they didn't listen."

"It's the way they are, I think it's the way they feel they have to be."

"So do I," said Sandra, who was a midwife herself. "That must change."

We talked for a while. "We'll be having another meeting soon," I said and I asked her to bring photos of her baby with her. She said she would. I told her that the other women were not upset when she was pregnant at the last meeting. They understood; they were really pleased for her.

"I met a woman who was a midwife at the Lourdes recently. She told me Neary removed her womb too. She said she begged him not to do it. But he still did it. Maybe I shouldn't tell people that?" Sandra asked.

"Of course you should. It's always harder for people in

the profession when something goes wrong, because they have a bigger hurdle to get over. The basis of their working lives are questioned as well."

"Yes, that's right," Sandra said. After a minute or two we signed off.

Later in the evening Niamh rang. I told her we had got on well. I explained that this was an investigation into whether there should be an investigation, that the committee was going to invite the hospital and Neary to appear before it, to be fair to all sides before they made up their mind, but they would probably not hold it now because of all the ongoing cases. There were circles within circles, legal cases within legal cases – civil, Medical Council, Oireachtas committees. I told Niamh that I totally believed we would get there in the end. There was no stopping the stone rolling.

Niamh spoke to me about her own legal case. I explained the several steps in the process as best I could. She, like most of the women, were naturally worried about taking legal action. In general, her solicitor explained that there are a number of specific steps that must be taken in an action for medical negligence. It is a long and arduous process for everyone involved. Niamh's case had reached the statement of claim stage.

By this time, in 2001, about sixty to sixty-five cases were proceeding along this path, with most of them at the statement of claim stage or earlier. One or two were at a more advanced stage and hoped to reach court by the end of the year.

Nicola rang too. "James got on grand. And there was no great bust-up."

"He didn't hit him, then?" I laughed. "That's great. I'm sure he feels better for having his say."

"He's a different man than left home. James says he did well. He identified our friend like a criminal in a line-up. Job done."

And Cathriona read over her statement of claim to me. Dr Neary was being sued for assault, battery and deceit.

Jim Reilly and I met Celia and her husband Patrick in Bewley's Hotel, one week to the day after the JOCHC meeting. Celia had had her womb removed by Neary in the early nineties.

Celia was looking lovely and was scented with some light perfume. Patrick looked like a film star in his suit, tall, tanned and fit, the image of a modern-day Errol Flynn. This was an important meeting for Celia and Patrick. They had missed the meeting when the NEHB had apologised to the women and their families for what had happened to them. They needed to meet with the official who attended that meeting. Jim was glad to oblige. We were taking him up on the offer to meet any of the women if that was needed.

Patrick asked Jim, "How high are you in the Health Board?"

"I'm the Senior Administrative Officer in the CEO's office."

Patrick nodded. He was satisfied.

"How did it all come out in the beginning?"

Jim told the facts, as he had told the November 1999 meeting with the group where the apology was presented.

"Will he ever practise again?"

"I don't think so," Jim said.

As Jim was speaking, I watched Celia's eyes become

heavy with sadness. They looked as if they were too heavy for her, as if their weight would make them slide into the back of her head.

"Celia is very, very sad about what happened to her. She was very sick after what happened," I said.

"I never believed these things happen in Ireland. You hear them about England but now I know they happen here too. I've known since this happened to Celia," Patrick explained to us.

"Anything that can happen has happened in Drogheda," said Jim, "but it will never happen again there, I can assure you of that."

"It's not just the NEHB; it's the whole country. We must make sure it doesn't happen anywhere in the whole country," I interjected. "The Medical Council will either throw the book at him or refer it to the guards."

We spoke about the Medical Council and its investigation. Celia expected to be going there to give evidence.

"They have the powers of a court. They can subpoena people to give evidence," Jim explained. "They're talking to anaesthetists at the moment. The solicitors are also considering referring their files to the police after the civil cases are over. Everything is slow, but we will get there."

"We will look after you when you are talking to the Medical Council. I'll meet you that morning," I said.

"You might like to meet one of the women who were already there before you go," suggested Jim.

Celia nodded quietly, saying yes. She is better by now and Patrick's anger is melting away. He trusts Jim.

"He won't be able to call himself doctor, I hope, after the Medical Council is finished its hearings," Celia commented.

"Butcher Neary, I call him," Patrick said.

"What about the 'the wise men'; do they exist?" Patrick asked. This is what all the women call the three obstetricians who wrote the report exonerating Neary.

"Oh, indeed they do," Jim said. "And three well-known obstetricians they are too. Very high profile. Very respected. The details of their report is under lock and key in our offices. In the safe."

"Is it true that Neary and Shine had their rooms beside each other in Drogheda?" I asked Jim, referring to the other scandal in the hospital.

"In Fair Street, yes. They have their private rooms there. There is a row of big houses on the street with cottages across from them. The doctors have their rooms in them. I'm not sure if they were immediately next door but they were near each other. Sure, they were great buddies. They were trying to buy Drogheda hospital from the nuns when it came up for sale, along with another doctor. But the NEHB got it."

"Oh, that doesn't bear thinking about," I said.

"Who is Shine?" asked Patrick.

"He's another doctor there who is up on charges of interfering with boys."*

"That's up for mention tomorrow in the Circuit Court," Jim told us.

"What's he charged with?" Patrick wanted to know.

"Indecent assault of teenage boys," I said.

"It won't be heard until about November," said Jim.

---

*Michael Shine was eventually acquitted of criminal charges of indecent assault, but was subsequently struck off the medical register by the Medical Council for professional misconduct.

Patrick and Celia were amazed. These injured people could still be shocked. Patrick was shaking his head from side to side, disbelief on his face.

We chatted around it all again. Having finished the tea, Celia and I gathered up our handbags and prepared to get up and go. Jim asked me to stay behind.

"We are going to the JOCHC next Thursday," he told me after Celia and Patrick had left.

"Who is going?"

"Me, Ambrose and the CEO. John Hamilton has been on to me."

I told him which TDs and senators were there.

"I'll let you know how we get on next week," he said.

I was mesmerised at the thought of Neary and Shine owning a hospital. I slept on that thought. I browsed through *The Irish Times* after breakfast. A columnist said he was not in favour of free health care because nothing is free in this world. He conceded that there was "something grotesque" about a seriously ill old lady needing help from the St Vincent de Paul Society to obtain crucial hospital care but said consultants should run their own private hospitals. I think, like Shine and Neary wanted to. I wondered why they wanted to buy Drogheda – to do more of the same, or was it fear they would get caught if someone other than the nuns ran it? Which was it? Who knows? Did it matter now? It mattered very much.

In early July, John Hamilton rang to say that the JOCHC were very interested in holding an investigation but could not, their legal advice was telling them, until the civil cases were over. I understood from him that this was a constitutional issue.

"Does the Medical Council investigation not interfere with matters then?" I asked.

"No."

"Well, that is good news."

John told me he would be putting this in writing. I was heartened. Every little helps.

11

More Straight Talk

Tony set up a meeting between Patient Focus and the Medical Council, so that the Council could get some exposure to the patients' views of how it did its business. On the day, 5 July 2001, Tony could not come to the meeting. I went with Cathriona, Noreen and Niamh. They wanted to tell the Council what it felt like to go through the process of complaining about a doctor, how the Council treated those who complained and the effect it had on them and their families. We were not going to speak of the ongoing inquiry in any way. We emphasised that to each other before the meeting.

We sat on one side of the long polished table in the Council boardroom. Members of the Council sat opposite us. The Council introduced themselves. Most of their names escaped me. I did catch that one was President of the Council, another was a psychiatrist, others were the lay members, including Dr Abdul Bulbulia, whose name I knew.

The President opened the meeting, formally welcoming us to the Council. I thanked them for agreeing to meet us.

"We want to listen and hear what you have to say," he said.

"Do you understand the functions of the Council?" the psychiatrist asked as he eyeballed me across the table and leaned forward. He was taking charge. I kept his gaze. "The Council's functions are very wide and include training and education. It's not just fitness to practise," he said.

I interrupted him. "Most people don't know of the Council's fitness to practise function. At a recent meeting we had, only one of about forty people knew of the existence of the Council, let alone fitness to practise," I said. "And people who do complain are very unhappy with the response they get. There are bad doctors like there are bad teachers, policemen, lawyers, but there is a reluctance to believe this, among the general population as well as among doctors." I was responding in kind.

"The fact that the Council is so unavailable to patients that were hurt contributes to the need people have to consult solicitors. The secrecy of the Medical Council perpetuates this," I went on. "Patients write in, they may or may not get a reply, very legally written, designed more to say what the Council can't do as opposed to what they can do. Mostly they are told there is no prima facie case. No one who gets this letter feels they have been listened to, that their complaint has been taken seriously. Neither would you in a similar situation." The women agree. That is their experience.

Then the President realises the people in front of him had ongoing cases. "The proceedings might be considered contaminated by this meeting," he said. We were asked to leave. "We will arrange another meeting," they said.

161

I said I did not agree with their analysis. The women were there in their capacity as members of Patient Focus, not as litigants. Dr Bulbulia wore two hats while he sat on the Council – he was a doctor and a lay member. Why couldn't the women?

However, I accepted that they made the decision in good faith. They would arrange another meeting very soon. I gave them my mobile number; they would definitely ring me the next day, they said.

We left, frustrated and upset.

"They didn't want to listen or hear what we had to say," said Noreen.

"Their body language was bad. They wanted us out," said Cathriona.

"They would rather not know," said Niamh.

"I think the lay members were listening and sympathetic," someone said.

I rang Niamh the next day.

"Did you tell Tony about yesterday?"

"I'll wait until he gets home."

"Yeah. We had good news anyway yesterday," Niamh said. "My cousin had a little girl. She had a caesarean, but everything is all right. I'm going in to see her this afternoon."

"That's great." I tried to keep the sorrow out of my voice. Back to the same hospital! My heart was sinking for Niamh. She was my friend. So was her mother.

I rang Tony at his surgery the following Monday and explained what had happened – that I was "provocative rather than aggressive", in my view.

"You have to be provocative. Otherwise no one will hear," he said.

"Thanks for that, Tony. Maybe I will have better luck with Deirdre Gillane, Micheál Martin's advisor, this afternoon. She phoned and suggested we meet to put faces on each other and fill each other in on developments."

In Jury's Hotel I spotted a woman I imagined might be the Minister's advisor in the corner of the foyer. She was reading documents and had a briefcase. In her thirties, I estimated, blonde, tall, athletic and pleasant-looking.

I asked if she was waiting for me. When she said yes, I sat beside her. I declined an offer of tea or coffee. Not because I'd just had some but because I didn't want to be a nuisance and interrupt things. She might be in a hurry.

"Water, then?"

"Water would be fine."

Deirdre came back in seconds with water and two glasses. Just what was needed, as it turned out.

I felt in no way rushed. I filled her in on the facts – how the information about Neary became public; how I got involved, radio, phone calls, the number of women in the group, meetings; how we helped put people in touch with legal and medical advice; how we had visited most if not all major politicians in the country; how everyone in Leinster House must know of us by now.

She had the "Whitewash Report" in front of her. "Even his colleagues were quite critical," she said, pointing to the report.

"Yes. And it's got much worse since then. The women need an independent public inquiry and a tribunal of compensation." Deirdre was writing notes on this.

"Are there many civil cases?"

"Over sixty-five at the moment."

"Who is being sued?"

"In the main, Dr Neary, but others too – the NEHB, the nuns, other professionals. Another problem is the large number of missing files. Damaged women whose files are missing can't prove their stories. They must be compensated in the light of what happened to others and in the knowledge of it. As well as that there are people who are emotionally unable to go to court. It would cause too much stress. Some people haven't even told their mother what happened to them."

Deirdre wrote again when I said that at least ten per cent of files were irretrievably lost. She asked about the response of the NEHB. I told her we thought it had been very supportive, paying for medical and other care for the women and their families.

"The Department of Health hasn't been great, though." I felt like emphasising this. "Contact has been very poor since the Minister came to Drogheda . Every time I ring it is a different civil servant who is dealing with it. There is no continuity. And the information they gave Mary Harney recently was at least four months out of date. We find it alarming that the Tánaiste does not get up-to-date information from the Department of Health. We knew more about it. Much more."

"That is why I am here," Deirdre said.

"Yes, and I am really pleased about that. The women are very disappointed in the Minister's decision not to set up an inquiry into the hospital until after the Medical Council reaches a verdict. They keep shifting their estimate of the date of a decision three months at a time. First they said

February, then June, now it's the autumn. But it won't happen in the autumn either because they are due to hear more witnesses then. It will be next June at the very earliest, or probably June 2003 or 2004. And they are so secretive, it's unbelievable. The women don't think it proper that the Medical Council can delay an inquiry in that way. Some delay is understandable, but not an indefinite one. Maybe the Minister could use this as a lever to action by the Medical Council. If the Medical Council delay is prolonged then we think the Minister should set up an inquiry anyway."

"That's reasonable," she said. "I tried to get information from them four times in the last fortnight with no luck."

"They asked us to leave. Threw us out last week," I told her, "on the grounds that they can't talk to the people who are involved in any particular ongoing case. You'd accept this if they were helpful in other ways, but they aren't. They just don't acknowledge any right of the public or the patient to have an opinion on how they do their business. They interpret the law in as restrictive a way as possible. They are secretive and call it confidentiality. It is not necessary at all." I tell her about how they didn't tell the women the location of the hearing on 16 October until the working afternoon before.

"Can the Minister get legal advice about their interpretation of the Medical Practitioners Act by the Medical Council? And find out what his options are? There must be something he can do."

"Yes, I can do that. I'll ask the legal advisor in the Department."

"Great."

"I'll get back to you on that."

"That's great."

"You can write to the full Council too," she said, "a personal letter to each council member."

"We will probably do that."

"In the meantime, you have a direct channel now."

"Yes. That will make an awful difference," I said as we shook hands and left.

I spoke to Tony later in the evening and told him about Deirdre Gillane, and what Cathriona and the other women thought. He told me the President of the Council was Professor Gerard Bury.

Tony was feeling bad that he hadn't been there. I emphasised that nothing untoward happened in the sense that people didn't shout at us or us at them. It was mannerly in its clinical way. In its coldness.

"I wouldn't have let them do that, put you out. I think we will have another go," Tony said. "This time just you and me." I agreed.

Later I spoke to Nicola. "I don't think I'd go through the Medical Council hearing again."

"Too painful?"

"Yes. I felt like I was nothing. And Neary sitting looking at you. Left to go out onto the street on your own after everything."

"Nicola, I will tell them all that when Tony and I go." I hear my voice lowering in sadness for Nicola and her husband.

"That's the truth," she said.

Afterwards I thought about this. I remembered how Nicola's letter was probably one of the issues that resulted in

Neary's suspension; in preventing him practising medicine pending an inquiry. I would tell her that the next time we spoke. Something really good did come from her actions, out of her very clear and detailed letter. I would remind her of that, of the women she saved.

On 23 July, *The Irish Times* carried a report by their political correspondent, Mark Hennessy, on the JOCHC investigation. This report included some details of the NEHB submission as to how the story came to their attention, how the health board reacted, etc. It also referred to Patient Focus calling for a full independent public inquiry into the hospital. A similar report appeared in the *Drogheda Independent* on 25 July. We were worried about this apparent leak of what we had understood to be confidential hearings.

In the following days I received anonymous phone calls accusing me of deliberately leaking confidential documents to the press. Tony was also receiving early morning phone calls from "the Drogheda ladies", saying they were going to set up a website in support of Neary. I was so concerned by the tone of these calls that I spoke to my local gardaí.

Jim got nuisance letters, accusing him of the leak and of wanting to close the hospital. "It's the last thing we want to do. We are pumping money into it. It's obviously a political leak; people with agendas. All I'm surprised about is that it took so long. Even the *British Medical Journal* has been on to us, asking if sixty-five women are suing."

On 3 August the formal letter from the JOCHC arrived. I was in the middle of painting the walls of our utility room at the time, but I stopped to read the mail in the envelope marked "Oireachtas". John Hamilton, at the request of the chairman, Mr Batt O'Keeffe, wrote that:

> *The Committee has been advised that the extent to which it could inquire into the practice of obstetrics and gynaecology would be severely limited while legal proceedings are ongoing. The Committee therefore decided to defer further consideration of this issue until court proceedings by the women involved against the consultant in question and the hospital has concluded.*

The committee thanked me for bringing this serious matter to their attention.

12

Drogheda Matrons

It was 15 August, the third anniversary of the Omagh bombing. The sun shone as I drove to Drogheda.

"People in Drogheda hospital have blood on their hands," Emily, one of the women in our group, had said to Mary Duff, the Director of Nursing in the Lourdes the previous week. This immediately resulted in an invitation from the Director to meet her at the hospital – another way to try and let the hospital know the women's feelings. Emily was not sorry but wondered if maybe she had spoken too strongly. She had been angry and said what was inside.

"No," I said. "Otherwise people won't get the message." She agreed. But we were pleased at Mary Duff's interest.

I arranged to meet Emily at the Europa Hotel at 3.00 p.m. We had an hour to discuss strategy. We arrived together and sat down to a pot of tea and home-made scones. We had the reception to ourselves, sitting on a couch at the door leading to the garden on this beautiful summer's day. Emily looked very elegant, blonde hair swept behind one ear, a side-parting, brown trousers, leather fitted jacket, white lace blouse. Lovely perfume.

We talked about our approach, about the need for a broader meeting in October to which Tony and the hospital's general manager would come.

Emily led the way to the hospital. We found it difficult to find places to park.

"They can wait a little while for us." Emily didn't like this place. "It makes the hairs stand on the back of my neck," she said as we walked in the front door. But she knew where she was going and why.

When we found the Director of Nursing's office, she was waiting for us. We were about ten minutes late.

"Colette McCann will be down in a moment. She was here a little while ago but I sent her back while we awaited your arrival. She worked for a long number of years in the maternity unit," Mary Duff said. Colette, we assumed, was the Assistant Director. We had heard her name mentioned by the women. "Sheila, you know Colette. She's on the midwifery committee with you."

"Yes, I know her, to see anyway. I haven't been to the meetings since last Christmas because I thought I was not getting anywhere."

"Were you not?" she seemed surprised.

"No. Maybe this isn't the time to talk about it," I said.

Colette arrived, a tall, pale-skinned, slender woman of fortyish. We shook hands and greeted each other.

Emily's manner was intimate as she opened the meeting. She didn't believe the ethos of Drogheda had changed since her painful experience there, when two nurses had commented casually on her scan. "There's nothing there," one had said to the other with a shrug of her shoulder. That was how Emily had found out she had lost her precious baby. She had to use a public phone to ring her husband with the news. No one would tell her what "ectopic" meant.

"The doctor, Neary, came in and said, 'I'll remove your tube this afternoon.' It was as if it was an exhaust pipe," she said.

A nurse had also told her, "Dr Neary might remove your ovary but he'll only do it if it is absolutely necessary." She had added, "He's the best."

That's the story Emily told the senior nurses at this meeting. The four of us sat around the teak-like table in the plain-looking office. Emily leaned forward as she spoke and looked them in the eyes. The Director blushed. She had never worked in the maternity unit.

Emily's skills at questioning were pivotal here. She was a star. Her message could not be avoided.

"I'm not saying you knew, but *people* knew," she said. "Why did nobody say anything?"

"Midwives were trained to say nothing. We were all trained that way. Doctors knew best. You dare not question them," Mary Duff explained.

"Yes, we all understand that, but it's not just enough to get rid of the bad egg; the culture that allowed it happen continues," Emily said, adding, "An infection still stays simmering. That must be eradicated."

"That's true, but all the staff here are very hurt," the Director said.

"I know," I chipped in. "I saw the reaction when I suggested our group meet the direct entry group. But they must feel the pain if any real change is to occur. Refusing to meet the women is self-protection. Refusing to take what happened on board. The women have had to face facts, their families, husbands, daughters, sons, mothers. What about the wonderful young girl who had her womb removed at nineteen? What about the girl who was just twenty, blonde like my twenty-year-old? I can't imagine how they feel but people are amazingly forgiving. All that has to be taken on board by the staff here if the culture is to change."

Emily said, "Explain to me how a midwife can complain here now. Explain to me how things are different."

"We have weekly meetings where everything is discussed."

"Yes, but has the culture changed enough that people are free to talk? The women believe it hasn't. That's what I hear," Emily stated.

"Is that what people say by word of mouth?" asked the Director.

"Yes," Emily said, "and there was subconscious knowledge of what happened in the hospital. An anaesthetist asked one woman after her caesarean hysterectomy if she noticed anything unpleasant in the theatre at the time. She hadn't. She was asleep. That person *knew* something. Perhaps she was hoping to have it confirmed by the patient to enable her to do something about it. Maybe she wanted to do something about it. And what can a woman do if she has a difficulty in here? That's the real issue." There seemed to be no clear-cut answer to this.

"People are well able to complain now," the Director said.

"I don't think they are," Emily said. "Some are but many are not."

"We can talk about this when we meet with Tony in October with the General Manager. We need a complaints scheme for the whole hospital. We don't know where this whole matter will end up," the Director of Nursing said.

"That's true," Emily agreed.

"Even now we feel we can answer any questions about how we have reacted when the whole Neary scandal broke." We agreed and knew Mary Duff was part of that. "We want to be a centre of excellence," she continued.

"Of course, it should be the whole hospital that takes this on board. Dr Shine is accused of abusing teenaged boys here. Some of them have contacted Patient Focus. It's not just the maternity unit," I said.

"Have they?" the Director asked.

"I don't think Drogheda is a hell-hole any more than other hospitals," I said.

"Oh, I know you don't, and it isn't."

"Things like this can happen in any hospital."

"And they do."

"We need a blueprint for how these things should be prevented and sorted."

"That's what we must get; we must get an inquiry," Mary Duff said.

I feel myself believing this woman, Mary Duff, the Director of Nursing. She wanted to meet us. She came to the meeting in the Boyne Valley, too. Colette McCann said little. She spoke only when spoken to but blood seemed to be reaching her face now. Her features had softened.

"It was a huge bereavement for all the people in our group," I said. "Some of the women in our group will never get over what happened. It is with them every second of every day."

"Is it?" the Director asked quietly.

I felt at last we were talking to whole people here. Hearts were opening. By now two hours had passed. It was time to end up. We made arrangements for Emily, Tony and me to come in October. Emily and I were pleased with this.

"I think we got through to them, do you?" she asked as we returned to our cars.

"Yes, I do, for the first time ever. Not just banging my head off a stone wall. Not just knocking on the door of an empty house. The lights are on but there is someone at home this time. Hearts have been prised open at last."

On the journey home I reflected that we must learn from history, otherwise we would repeat it. The people in the hospital wanted to protect themselves from pain – the pain of the truth. They understood each other's pain; they were much less able to understand the damaged patient's pain. That damage can happen is everyone's fault. That it does is the fault of the perpetrator. They had to let in the pain if anything was to be learned from this. The institutional "monster" of all the blind eyes and deaf ears had to be recognised and faced down.

By mid-September we still had no word from Deirdre Gillane in the Minister's office, and we were waiting to hear from Mary Duff, the Director of Nursing, about our meeting on 18 October.

"Maybe they were not opening up like we thought. Maybe they were just momentarily undone like a zip in an embarrassing place, quickly zipped up again," I said to Emily when she called to ask if I had heard anything. "But RTÉ have been in touch in the last few days. They are thinking of doing a *Prime Time* documentary about Drogheda and Neary. Mary Raftery is the producer involved and I told the researcher Sheila Ahern the whole story."

In mid-October, Mary Duff rang about the next meeting. "You're a hard woman to get," she told me. "I rang a few times and the phone rang out." I knew she was right; I could be hard to get. I had been unfair to Mary in thinking she had changed her mind about the meeting. Clearly she hadn't and was acting on her promise to Emily and me.

"How many women were you thinking of bringing? Dr Lynch and Dr Milner here will be there, along with nurse managers from here," Mary began.

I was very pleased that they were willing to meet the women. "Oh, we weren't thinking of bringing any women at this stage, only Tony, Emily and myself. I think the women is for the longer term. The much longer term, over two or three years. I'm sorry, I didn't mean to cause that misunderstanding."

"I'm happy about that," she said, "because many people here are not ready for that yet either."

"Same with the women," I said. "It would be awful if that didn't go well. A lot of thought must go into that. An awful lot."

"I'm relieved to hear you say that. I've not been the flavour of the month here for some time." I knew this woman was trying her very best.

"I'm sure. I understand how difficult it can be for everyone. The hospital too. I'm not out to destroy anyone. I couldn't live with myself if it made anyone unable to cope. I thought the meeting in August was very intense. I understand these things are very difficult all round."

"The culture is much different here now from then," she said. "There are contacts with other hospitals now and with other departments. Things are much different."

"That's good," I said.

"Women who come in here now for their third or fourth baby say it is very different than before," Mary said.

"Of course, and I'm sure it's true, but the women who were hurt matter. They are not out for vengeance, they are not looking for a blood-letting. They just need to know that things have changed. That will really help them."

"Will it?"

"Yes, of course, and it has already. The meeting you and Jim and Sally came to mattered. But they need to know that the changes go down to the people who do the day-to-day work. They see the change in management. They would love to see the change in the nursing and medical staff too. That's what this is all about. We won't be forcing anyone on either side to get involved in it. But it would be a great help."

She suggested a date for the meeting.

Niamh rang next morning. I tell her Cathriona has just suggested we set up a meeting with local politicians. She thinks this is a great idea and offers to contact the TDs in North Dublin. I tell her too of the meeting at the hospital, and of the nuisance phone calls, which continue. They seemed designed to prove that I had a malevolent purpose to my work.

"Don't mind them, they're just nuts," she said.

"And how is your little girl?" I ask.

"She's great. She's mad."

"She's at that age," I said.

"She had her birthday a few days ago. Do you want to talk to her?"

Niamh's little girl told me of her bouncy castle and her party. How I wasn't there when she was three, as if everyone in the world was at her party.

"Next time," she said.

"Next time," I promised.

Tony and I met Emily at the Europa Hotel, on our way to the Lourdes Hospital for the long-planned and anticipated meeting with the maternity unit staff. On arrival Mary Duff and Dr Maura Milner, a newly recruited obstetrician, were there. We waited a couple of hours, hoping against hope that someone else would come. But nobody else came. We spoke to Mary and Maura anyway.

"I am really sorry for bringing you all this way," Mary said, apologising for the failures of others. "It must be because they have been subpoenaed to appear before the High Court. It's probably legal advice. Many tears have been shed here in this unit about this. People here are hurting. They were afraid they would break down."

"We have all cried," Emily said as one of the women and on behalf of the others.

"The staff have concerns about the money Patient Focus got from the NEHB too. There's talk about it in the hospital. I didn't know about that either." Mary was trying to explain the absence.

"Because we only got it very recently, and it's the first money Patient Focus got. It just covers stamps, phones and hiring of hotel rooms for meetings," I explained. "Tony and I have been covering phones and stamps ourselves."

"My staff never had counselling either. They were offered it but they never took it up. The women have been looked after," Mary said.

"I hope they are not so selfish as to equate what happened to the women to the situation they are in," I said.

In the lift leaving the hospital we agreed to try again after Christmas.

"The zip has been fully closed now," Emily said as we travelled home. "The staff are not going to go there. The message is not getting through. It probably never will." We had to agree.

"The question of our money from the NEHB is a total red herring, too. I am getting loads of nuisance phone calls. I've put the phone down on so many people recently, each giving me a different name, accusing me of all sorts, being out to destroy the wonderful Dr Neary. I had to ask Colm to send one of them a solicitor's letter last week, threatening an injunction and a complaint to the gardaí."

"What a waste of an evening," Tony said again when we got back to Dublin. "And isn't it just as well we didn't bring more of the women? It would have been totally terrible."

On Thursday 29 November, I attended the launch in the Mansion House Round Room of the government's new Health Strategy. A room with a ceiling speckled with stars. It was a bright, crisp morning. My mood was similar.

A friend kept a place for me – second row from the front. I really appreciated that. No copies of the strategy were provided. "It won't be available until after the presentation," my friend explained. "Stops people asking awkward questions."

Despite the beautiful ceiling in this room, the sky was not the limit for change. Not in mindsets anyway. It was very difficult to break down defences. I thought this after we had been thrown out of the Medical Council in July. And again after the meeting with the nurses in October in Drogheda. And now the Medical Council are not returning Tony's calls about a rescheduling of that fiasco.

Deirdre Gillane rang, though, but only after I made efforts to get the press interested. Legal advice prevented the Minister taking action to hurry up the Medical Council, she told me. Everything I said was true. She knew it. I knew it. What she said was true too. We were learning to wait.

Everyone in that round room seemed different from me. They lived in a world where medicine was always good. They were not as safe as they thought. It is mostly the old who have degrading contact with the health service. But it happens to others too. A young woman giving birth: isn't that everyone? We needed quality care. We needed a complaints system We needed a change in the law governing the Medical Council to make it more transparent.

I listened to the wonderful presentation, the plans, proposals, and the congratulations to the Minister for his job well done. No mention here in this room of haemophiliacs, Brigid McCole or Neary. That was real. It didn't fit the Strategy presented in this lovely room. It fitted the dim lights, though. Let's look, but not too closely lest we see. I listened on, talked to nice people, ate a good lunch. It was 3.30 before I left and there were no copies of the Strategy left for me. Later in the week I found Tony had been and had kept one for me.

Part 3

Going Public

Valerie's Story

Valerie was a midwife in the hospital where her baby was delivered and where Dr Neary, her colleague and doctor, removed her womb. Her first pregnancy ended sadly with the death of the baby she was carrying. Dr Neary took excellent care of her during that pregnancy. I have not had the honour of knowing Valerie.

Valerie trained as a midwife in Drogheda and worked alongside Dr Neary and other consultants there. She told her story to the Fitness to Practise Committee of the Medical Council. She was pregnant with her second baby through 1996. She went into labour when she was five days overdue in August 1996. She made a little progress in her labour overnight and asked for an epidural. Dr Neary came in during the night and suggested an oxytocin drip. By morning, though, she was not ready to deliver her baby.

"I spoke to Dr Neary and he suggested I might consider a section and I consented," she told the committee. This was

decided at 11.00 or 11.10 a.m. and her baby was born shortly after at 11.50.

"Dr Neary took over the baby to make sure he was okay." Valerie was delighted with her new baby.

"Dr Neary came back over to the table and said I was bleeding quite heavily. He ordered a repeat of the syntocin to stop bleeding. He ordered hot packs as well. He said he was massaging my uterus too.

"I had realised there were a lot of hysterectomies being carried out at the hospital over the previous year and was beginning to panic. He turned around a couple of minutes later and said, 'I have to carry out a hysterectomy.'"

"No, you cannot," Valerie said.

"One of the midwives was crying. She was looking down with tears in her eyes."

A ward sister came in through the theatre doors. "Dr Neary, we will get Dr Lynch in," she said.

"He said there wasn't time; he would carry out a hysterectomy." Her baby was about six or seven minutes old at the time of this conversation between Neary and Valerie. "I said, 'Don't do a hysterectomy on me.'" She remembered his habit of performing hysterectomies. "I was sure there must have been something he could do to help me out. I did not feel as if my life was in danger."

"I had a bit of chest pain," Valerie said when Neary told her he needed to do a hysterectomy. It was stress.

"He never convinced me I needed it . . . I never gave consent," she said.

Valerie had two units of blood administered, one in theatre and another in recovery. She was back in recovery by 1.15 p.m. Dr Neary came into the recovery room and said he did all he could and he was sorry. *"I know he came to my room that evening to see how I was getting on but I could not talk to him."*

The following day, he told Valerie she had a large fault in her uterus. She had practically no muscle, he said, so there was nothing to contract and stop the bleeding. He said the surgery was necessary.

"He said it might have something to do with a drug my mother might have taken after one of her pregnancies." He also told her she was lucky to have kept her ovaries, as another doctor wanted to take them. She had to believe him, she said.

"Two years later, after a story in The Irish Times, *I asked for my pathology notes, to find out everything was normal."* (She did lose 1,500–2,000 ml of blood, according to Dr Neary's barrister at the inquiry, Mary Finlay.) Neary was found guilty of professional misconduct in Valerie's case.

13

Valerie's Case

Sheila Ahern and I met in the Four Courts
case. We waited for *Neary* v *Neary* to begi
in the Round Hall looked as if they
strangely different sect. Most dressed in
perched on top of their heads. Some of the
like tummies under waistcoats that act
railing them in. At least I'm wearing a
jacket, even if it is from Penney's. It's chee
Out of the corner of my eye I see a tall sli
neat urchin hair, long legs in a pin-stri
gown.

"Look at her," I said to Sheila Aher
dressed and still feminine."

"It's the pose," she said. "The way sh

"So it is not what you wear but h
replied.

he did all he could and he was sorry. "I know he came to my room that evening to see how I was getting on but I could not talk to him."

The following day, he told Valerie she had a large fault in her uterus. She had practically no muscle, he said, so there was nothing to contract and stop the bleeding. He said the surgery was necessary.

"He said it might have something to do with a drug my mother might have taken after one of her pregnancies." He also told her she was lucky to have kept her ovaries, as another doctor wanted to take them. She had to believe him, she said.

"Two years later, after a story in The Irish Times, *I asked for my pathology notes, to find out everything was normal."* (She did lose 1,500–2,000 ml of blood, according to Dr Neary's barrister at the inquiry, Mary Finlay.) Neary was found guilty of professional misconduct in Valerie's case.

185

13

Valerie's Case

Sheila Ahern and I met in the Four Courts for the first Neary case. We waited for *Neary* v *Neary* to begin. Nearly everyone in the Round Hall looked as if they belonged to some strangely different sect. Most dressed in black or with wigs perched on top of their heads. Some of the men have Rumpole-like tummies under waistcoats that act as a type of corset, railing them in. At least I'm wearing a baby-pink fleecy jacket, even if it is from Penney's. It's cheerful. It's warm too. Out of the corner of my eye I see a tall slim woman in black, neat urchin hair, long legs in a pin-striped trouser suit, a gown.

"Look at her," I said to Sheila Ahern. "The way she is dressed and still feminine."

"It's the pose," she said. "The way she stands."

"So it is not what you wear but how you wear it," I replied.

"Obviously."

Still the little groups huddled around like talking heads, whispering to one another. Behind Sheila and me was a group of people huddled together conspiratorially. One was jumping around excitedly, eyes bouncing as if on springs. One of his friends was very thin.

"They're here because the first Christian Brother civil abuse case starts today," I heard someone say.

In front of us are three barristers. I heard one say to the other, "They looked after the poor in the fifties. They educated everyone, regardless of financial means. It was just the times. Everyone was beaten."

"I wasn't," I said to Sheila, who was there as researcher for the *Prime Time* programme she was hoping to do on Neary.

"Most weren't," she said.

Sherwin v *Independent News Papers Ltd* was the only case blinking on the neon notice board, advertising its wares like Coca Cola.

We sat around on the brass bars of the round room, waiting for things to happen. We went in and out of Court No 1. It is here cases are allocated to specific judges.

The court registrar explained the delay to us. "There are no judges. They are trying to find some." As if the judges had been mislaid or lost in some way.

I recognised all sorts of people in this cathedral to the law. Still no case starts. "It's worth it, though," I said to Sheila. "It's like an orientation course. So I know where I am going and what to expect when I come with the women."

We went home and would come back the next day. The first Neary case still hadn't started. There was no sign of Neary yet.

All of the regular women phoned later.

"How did things go? How was Valerie?"

"No news to report yet," I said. Niamh rang. She would come tomorrow.

A windy day. I was blown about a bit as I made my way to the Four Courts. Sheila Ahern was there before me.

"It's been allocated a court – number 6."

"Ah, great."

I was looking around for Niamh. I recognised people from the day before: the men from the Christian Brothers case, some of the same old barristers. People stood around whispering, as if gossiping. People waited inside and out in this Round Hall. I saw Niamh and waved to her. She looked pale.

"Are you okay?"

"Yes, just walked from Parnell Square." She must have been asking herself how on earth she had ended up here. I asked myself how on earth she ended up here.

We found Court 6 after we asked directions from wandering barristers.

"How can you take someone seriously dressed like that?" I said to Niamh as we walked towards the courtroom door.

"It's meant to scare you," Niamh said.

"They don't have to wear them," Sheila said. "Better turn off our mobiles. Don't want to end up in jail."

We sat three rows from the back, three rows from the front. There were very few in the room. Barristers mumbling, shuffling, may-it-please-your-lordship types from *Kavanagh QC*. Highly polished bench seats like in a church, but with green padding. Cream walls, a fan blowing in the left-hand corner. Obviously it gets very hot in here. I heard a case being adjourned. A barrister came in, laden with files, placed them in front of us. A tall woman, very thin, came with a man. They made their way into the seat immediately in front of us. I knew it was Valerie Neary, even though she was not in our group. Niamh did too. What I assumed to be her family – mother and father, and sister or friend – sat next to her. A tall man in a pinstripe suit talked to the barrister about whatever was in the file they peered into. The nurses from the hospital filed in behind us. Valerie was a midwife in Our Lady of Lourdes Hospital. How strange she must have felt in this courtroom now. She would have been very welcome in our group. But everyone understood her need for privacy.

Two women were beside me. I was unsure of who they were at first. Then I recognised Colette McCann, the Assistant Director of Nursing at the Lourdes and Kathleen Lambe, who worked in its medical records office and was looking after the search for the women's records. We shook hands and Kathleen and I exchanged mobile numbers.

The couple in front went in and out once or twice. Then in again. Valerie turned around to us. "How did you know my case was on?" she asked me.

I said we were there to support her. We wished her luck and told her that all the women were thinking of her that morning and wishing her well. I hoped I was not too presumptuous, too cheeky.

She seemed pleased. A gentle, tired woman; pretty and dignified. Her husband smiled too, his arm round her. She was a midwife in the same unit; her colleagues were sitting behind me. Sadly, she would die soon. She had terminal cancer.

A court clerk opened the door to the left for the judge. "All rise," he said. He pulled out the big chair on the podium for the judge, who sat down.

Neary v *Neary* was called. Dr Neary, the defendant, was not there. His barrister rose. Gleeson was his name, Arthur Cox the solicitors. "The same solicitors who represented the Christian Brothers," Sheila told me.

"Just recently we have received additional pleadings re the Statute of Limitations," the barrister continued.

"It is in relation to a caesarean hysterectomy and a statement by the defendant about a defective fundus in my client's womb," Valerie Neary's barrister said. "We want to introduce evidence of a conversation between my client and the defendant."

"I want to do justice to all the parties here so do you not want to seek an adjournment?" the judge asked.

Michael Neary's barrister rose again. "There are special circum-stances here," he explained.

"To do with the defendant or the plaintiff?" asked the judge.

"The plaintiff," Gleeson replied, "we need to resolve this soon. Without giving you the full details, there is a significant illness involved."

"Would a break help?" asked the judge. "Twenty minutes?"

The barristers agreed it probably would.

"We will resume at twelve noon," the judge said.

"All rise."

I saw Valerie rise gingerly. She was very thin. She leaned back.

"This will be a difficult case to prove," she confided in us.

"Will it?" I asked. "We wish you luck."

We adjourned to the canteen, past the law library, down the stairs. Sheila bought us tea.

All were back again at noon. More time was needed; we adjourned until two. Sheila Ahern couldn't stay.

Niamh and I had lunch together in a little coffee shop with comforting scones. We sat by the window, looking out on the world. We talked, small talk for the most. I wondered what a lovely young girl like her was doing there.

"No one's the same after what happened to Valerie Neary," she said, meaning not just her but all the women.

"No, never the same. But at least after you recover you know you can cope with awful things. Most people don't know that. They think their world falls apart if they don't get what they want for Christmas."

"I used to be concerned about things like that. I wouldn't care now if I got nothing for Christmas," Niamh said.

We chatted away.

"I think I'll stay until it is over," I said. "Aideen, my kid, forgot her key. But she is able to open the door without it anyway. I'm staying."

"I'll stay until three, anyway. I'll see then," Niamh said.

I talked about Aideen

"She is nearly late for school every morning because she has started wearing make-up to school and it takes her about ten minutes but she still gets up at the same time as before."

"Do they wear makeup to school these days?" You would think Niamh had left school years earlier, the way she said that.

It was 1.45, time to be going back. In the courtroom the barrister rose.

"A settlement has been reached," he said. "It is without liability."

"I will write that into the records of the court," the judge said. He bent forward, pen in hand, and wrote. "I am very pleased this has happened in this case." And with that, he left.

"Is it over?" we asked ourselves.

It was all over. There was shaking of hands. All very civilised.

Valerie Neary was on the six o'clock news on RTÉ, talking to the reporter Mary Wilson. She was interviewed in her own sitting room, her husband beside her and her little boy's picture on the wall behind her, telling her story quietly and with enormous dignity. Valerie was wearing the same jumper as in the court earlier. She had not specially dressed up for TV. She looked relaxed, happy and safe now, if frail. She had lovely soft eyes that said everything.

And there Neary was, large as life, striding up the pathway on his way in the door of Lynn House on 16 October 2000.

For the rest of the evening my phone didn't stop ringing, woman after woman saying how wonderful they thought her, how they cried as she talked, how young she looked, how grateful they were to her. There was hope and relief in their voices because it was all coming out at last. There was a hint of "almost too good to be true" there as well. They had been afraid to hope but could do so now at last. They wanted to thank her.

Tony rang too. I said I was considering sending Paul Maguire an email asking him to read out a thank you from the women to Valerie.

"That's a great idea," he said.

"Do you feel proud of yourself tonight, Tony?"

"Yes," he said.

"And so you should," I said. We spoke about the lack of courage of some other doctors, those unable to do the right thing.

"It is fear of the profession," he said.

"We all have our fears. It's a lack of character that stops us doing the right thing in situations like this," I said.

"It is."

Tony didn't want to get off the phone. He was happy to muse, to taste the sense of relief that we were absolutely, definitely, unquestionably on the right side. To digest the sense of wellbeing that comes from having done the unpopular right thing. Because it was very unpopular among Tony's closest and oldest friends.

The phone continued to ring. The different tone to the women's voices was only too obvious: hope, vindication at last, public recognition, energy reawakened to conquer grief. I think my voice was different too.

I sent the email to Paul Maguire of LMFM asking him to thank Valerie on air for her courage in going public. His response said it all: "Only too happy to oblige."

The local radio station was trying to track down Valerie. I didn't have a number for her but told them her solicitor's name. They wanted to know if I could get a couple of the women to talk live on the show. For the first time I knew I could ask them, safe in the knowledge that they would now be able to do it. I rang Niamh first. She told me she couldn't, that she hadn't got that far yet. Nicola said yes; Noreen said yes. Cathriona would have done it, so too would Jenny. No shortage of people, all ready to tell it now. No more heads down. It was walking tall from now on, out in the light, in the sunshine that was shining despite the December day. After Valerie Neary, the other women were able to talk. That is what she did for them.

I couldn't get LMFM in Dublin so I didn't hear Valerie. But I heard Nicola and Noreen because I was on the phoneline to the show at the time. I felt pleased and stunned that we had got to that point. Noreen spoke of the importance of the recognition of their suffering and the need for a public inquiry. Nicola said she wanted Neary to admit he did wrong, to come out with his hands up and to admit all the lies. He had told her she was the first; that he had saved her life instead of destroying it.

It was all over. The boil had been lanced. Noreen and Nicola rang me within five minutes of getting off the radio. They were both fine, both proud of themselves. How far Nicola and I had come since that first meeting in the Boyne Valley Hotel. Noreen was always a spirited and dignified lady. Always.

That afternoon, Susan McKay of the *Sunday Tribune* got in touch. "I've just been talking to Valerie Neary for an article this Sunday. I understand you are involved with the group?"

"Yes. I'm the group's co-ordinator, I suppose."

"I was wondering, could I put a contact number at the end of the piece? Tony O'Sullivan's or yours. And maybe an email address. Would that be okay?"

"Of course."

"Valerie is very forgiving. She doesn't think there was anything malicious," Susan said.

"That's right. Two women in our group were on the radio with her this morning and that's what they said."

"I got a shiver up my spine listening to her speak, as if there was something sinister going on, the way she said she asked him to stop and he didn't."

"I sometimes get that feeling listening to the women too. Now nearly everyone thinks there was something sinister going on, especially the men and most of the women. It's hard not to think that."

"I need to get this off so that it will be published on Sunday. Are you sure it's all right about the contact numbers?"

"Yes, of course, those numbers are out there in public anyway."

About five minutes later, Susan rang again.

"There seems to be much more to this than I thought. I am very interested in it. Can we talk some time?"

We decided on the following Wednesday.

The women loved Susan's article on Sunday 10 December. The headline was: "LYING ON THE TABLE, I COULD DO NOTHING. I WAS POWERLESS. I SAID, DON'T DO IT". The subheading read, "Midwife Valerie Neary was forced to have a hysterectomy she did not want or need".

The article told how staff at the hospital knew there was a very high caesarean hysterectomy rate there. How Valerie asked her husband not to let Neary do a hysterectomy if he put her to sleep. How she knew her vital signs were fine and she was in no danger. How her colleagues wanted to get a second opinion but Neary said there wasn't time. How he told her she was lucky she didn't lose her ovaries and how Valerie knew that was rubbish. How the excuses he gave her were exactly the same as he gave to the other women. He denied these excuses, yet I had heard it all before.

I felt very sad, shocked even, after reading the article. It made it truer still. No one wants to believe these things happen.

14

The Neary Support Website Strikes

"Mum, come here! Have you seen the Neary website recently? It's been updated."

Aideen came out of the office, a hint of hysteria in her voice, just days before Christmas. "There's loads of stuff about you and Tony O'Sullivan on a Neary website."

I'd been feeling very sorry for myself. I'd had a tummy bug for days. It was particularly bad that morning. I was feeling exhausted and all I wanted to do was watch the Christmas edition of *Brookside*. The last thing I wanted to do was engage my brain. However, adrenalin is a powerful hormone. I was already by Aideen's side, looking over her shoulder at the screen. She scrolled up and down. Key words leapt out at me like "kicks", "Medical Council", "report", "FOI", "Dept of Health", "collusion", "sex scandals".

"They're going to report Tony to the Medical Council – look." Aideen pointed out more.

"They've released the letters I wrote to Micheál Martin including the September 2000 one.* Surely that should be protected? They have sent those letters to the maternity staff, the Irish Nurses Organisation, the Irish Medical Organisation and the Irish Hospital Consultants Association . . . What about the people in the hospital? We were just building up relationships again with the staff, the midwives. I'd better ring Tony and tell him."

I couldn't get him; the phone was engaged. I rang Cathriona. She knew from the tone of my voice that I was upset.

"What's wrong, Sheila?"

I told her. We talked on for a while about the next meeting, letters, that I'd been sick all week, Christmas. I felt a little bit better.

In a while I got through to Tony. I told him he is to be reported to the Medical Council for professional misconduct. He laughed.

"Then they won't be able to talk to me either." He was referring to the incident where we had been thrown out in July.

"Are you not worried?"

"Not really."

"I did run the September 2000 letter past Hugh Thornton before I sent it out. He described it as robust. But he said it would probably come under qualified privilege. You have to be able to do something about terrible things, otherwise no one could write anything of a serious nature about anything they were worried about."

The next morning I got in touch with Jim Reilly. He hadn't seen the website but he knew about the letter. He

---

*See letter on page 96

198

knew that senior people in the hospital got it too. The NEHB were sending it to their legal advisor. The hospital was not going to do anything about it.

"I can't find the letter on my computer but I remember it. I read it out to one of the solicitors before sending it off."

"It's a September one. We got a copy of it at the time."

"Oh yes, it's the one I wrote it after spending a weekend talking to the women after they met Dr Clements. Everything in it is true. The Department of Health handed over that letter without even telling me – not even a phone call. I told Tony as well that he is going to be reported to the Medical Council."

"I'm sure he's really worried!"

"Right enough, he didn't seem to care too much. I thought it would take the sleep of the night off me but it didn't. My husband is dead cool about it as well."

"Don't give up the cause now," he said.

I couldn't.

Next, I got on to Colm MacGeehin, our solicitor, after finding a copy of the September 2000 letter to Micheál Martin. I was alarmed by the honesty of the letter, the truthfulness of it. The directness. In a way I was proud of myself. I read it all out to Colm.

When I finished, he said, "It's all true; it was informed by the facts. Neary has no reputation now."

"But what about the other staff in the hospital?"

"That's fair comment from the facts," Colm said. "You have nothing at all to worry about. Forget it. Don't give it another moment's thought."

I phoned the Minister's project manager, Deirdre Gillane. She had time to talk. I told her what had happened. I read out the middle paragraph again. I said I was not informed it was to be released, that I would have expected to be. Can no one tell the truth without being totally exposed? What if you didn't have proof, only concerns or suspicion; can you not tell the Minister for Health?

Deirdre was sympathetic, but the Freedom of Information (FOI) section is independent of the Minister's office. "We have nothing to do with it. We can't. We wouldn't even know there was a request in," she said. But she was soothing.

I made my own enquiries. The phone was answered by a woman in the FOI section. She told me that Eddie Flood was dealing with that and she would transfer me to him. There was no answer from his extension. Eddie Flood sounded familiar. I looked up my contacts file. Denis O'Sullivan is his Principal Officer. I got on to him and told him my story. He sounded concerned. He could understand why I was upset.

I told my daughter Katie. As usual she asked why.

"If it's true, why can't you say? If they sue you, just tell them to piss off." She read the website pages I had printed off. "What's the problem anyway? They aren't even denying anything. They're admitting everything happened. The problem seems to be that it wasn't just Neary. That makes the whole thing even worse."

Then I remembered the conversation with Hugh Thornton, how he had said he was personally having difficulty coping with what Dr Clements said to him after he had seen the women. How it had affected him emotionally. How he found it difficult to believe this had happened in the Lourdes, and that there was another consultant there charged with indecent assault on teenage boys. How he would find it difficult to look at the women the next time he saw them. How he would do what he could do legally, including pursuing it in the criminal courts after the civil cases were over. How it was up to Tony and me to bring it to the attention of the politicians to ensure it never happened again. That was our role. Hugh was emotional. Hugh was right. So was Katie. So was Wilfie. So was Tony. So was I.

Over Christmas I wrote a letter to Mary Duff, the Director of Nursing in the Lourdes, and to Colette McCann, apologising if they were hurt in any way by the letter. I reassured them I had not sent it. I also asked Mary Duff to try to arrange another meeting for the women with staff members.

15

Persuasion

Before Christmas we invited all the local TDs to meet the women. The meeting was planned for January when the Dáil would be on Christmas holiday. There was an election due the following summer and we felt this was the time to approach the TDs in the four constituencies. Cathriona and I sent the invitations to the TDs in early December. We also wrote to the women, asking them to contact their local TDs to encourage them to come to the meeting. This ended up as a huge exercise in local democracy. Women phoned, wrote, cajoled their local representatives in an effort to persuade them to come to the meeting, which was as usual to be held in the Boyne Valley.

We were very keen to persuade Michael Bell to come, as he was the local Drogheda TD. We put special effort into persuading him. I even wrote to his party leader, Ruairi Quinn, in this regard.

At first the response from some of the TDs was non-committal. Many of them seemed to know very little of what had happened in the Lourdes.

"I've had very little luck," Maura told me down-heartedly. "It's very hard to interest them. The only one we're sure of is Trevor Sargent of the Greens."

I spoke to Deputy Nora Owen of Fine Gael and asked her to come to the meeting.

"Is this doctor still practising?" she asked.

I told her of the Medical Council inquiry and how they can take years. One had taken nine years so far and it was still not over. I told her too of the settlement in Valerie Neary's case before Christmas.

"There must be something to it," she said, "otherwise they wouldn't have struck him off. I'll ask around," she added, "before I make my mind up."

The TDs didn't want to come. They had to be made to by their constituents. The women phoned and phoned again, yet no one felt they were getting anywhere. We thought about calling off the meeting, but changed our minds.

I rang the Taoiseach's office and Michael Noonan's office and left messages asking them to encourage TDs to come. The lack of interest continued. Deputies offered to meet in the Dáil, take people for a drink, entertain even, but that was no good. There was a landslide of indifference everywhere. But the women kept phoning until their luck turned.

Nora Owen said she was coming. Sean Ryan of Labour was coming, so too was Caoimhghín Ó Caoláin of Sinn Féin and Seymour Crawford of Fine Gael. This was better than a Lotto win. The interest continued: Johnny Brady, Sean Farrelly; Mary Wallace was sending a representative. Noel Dempsey would be in China so he couldn't come. The tide had turned, though.

Nicola rang the Louth TDs. Seamus Kirk was only a maybe. "I argued with him," she said. "I wanted him to say yes but all he would say was 'if nothing else happens in the meantime'. I kept saying, 'What can be more important than this?' but he wouldn't give me a definite yes. So I take it as a no. But he might come yet."

"Yes, he probably will in the end."

"The Minister, Dermot Ahern. I rang him. The girl in the office asked immediately if I was from Patient Focus. So I said yes. She said he'd be there if he could." Brendan McGahon was coming too, she said.

"Oh, that's great."

"He's very direct."

"Yeah, I've seen him on television. He's a man who speaks his mind."

"I needed wellies to wade through the muck on the way into his office. I think he's retiring, too. He got on the phone to the NEHB while I was sitting in front of him. He said he was a friend of Ambrose McLoughlin's. He spoke to someone called Gerry. 'Tell me about this Neary fellow and Patient Focus,' he said. Then he went on that he had a woman sitting in front of him who didn't seem to be out of her mind, 'but I just wanted to check for myself'." Nicola was laughing as she told this story. "He said he'd come then and I said he'd better; then he barked, 'If I said I will then I will'. He knew me from where I worked. He used to come in every day."

"He'll come." I said. "This has worked brilliantly and one of the best things has been the way all the women have pulled this off. Even Sara rang yesterday after persuading Johnny Brady to come."

"And she used to get so upset.'

"One thing I know now for [...]
public inquiry and a tribunal o[...]
from Jim Reilly. Because wh[...]
Christmas he was afraid I w[...]
'You can't stop now, Sheila.' S[...]
you find out what people are thinking[...]

"Oh, you wouldn't, would you?" Nicola[...]

"There is no chance of that. There never was[...]
didn't know that and he was worried for a second."

"That's what we want," she said. "We can't stop until
we get it."

On Monday, 14 January, I think I got out of the bed on the
wrong side. Everything, everyone irritated. I badgered our
solicitor too.

"Oh God, Colm, I hope you will have a presentation
ready for Wednesday night. We spent the last eight weeks
setting this up, badgering people to come. This is our last
chance; all the politicians are coming; we won't get them all
in the same room again. Will you give the presentation?"

"I will, okay." He seemed, naturally enough, to be still
finding his feet after the weekend. "I've had the 'flu all last
week and I'm only just back today. It'll be ready, I'll do it this
evening with Senior Counsel and you'll have it tonight."

"That's great, oh thank God for that. And we need to be
ready to start at eight sharp."

"I know, politicians always want to be moving on."

"Yes they have places to go and people to see. Always
moving on to the next event."

"Don't worry, it'll be ready," Colm said.

d I was in, nothing would reassure me.

were still a couple more politicians to persuade. I
puty GV Wright again. I had phoned him at home
ght before and he had promised to see what he could
got back to him and he was still not clear. He had a
ection convention going on, he said,

The morning of the meeting Dermot Ahern's secretary
rang. "The Minister can't make the meeting tonight. He
sends his apologies."

"That's a pity," I said.

"The Minister is in touch with Micheál Martin frequently
and he is aware of the situation," she told me.

Wednesday arrived at last. Most of the politicians came:
Seamus Kirk, Johnny Brady, John Farrelly, Andrew Boylan,
Brendan McGahon, Seymour Crawford, John Bruton, Nora
Owen, Sean Ryan, Caoimhghín Ó Caoláin . . .

Michael Bell didn't, as far as we know. He didn't make
himself known to us anyway. Noel Dempsey never sent a
representative. Mary Wallace sent a representative. But as
Minister for Equality and Women's Affairs, we thought she
should have come herself.

Local councillors and senators and members of the
Health Board were all there. Each had to have their say. One
met his cousin there; he never knew she was one of Neary's
victims. Most were wholeheartedly supportive. Most were
shocked, or at least that's what they said.

The women spoke of their experiences, telling their
stories of buried grief. One woman told me quietly that
evening that it was as if Neary had physically occupied her
body and slept in it for twenty years. Hidden there, a serpent

asleep within her. It was a make-or-break moment for her, she said. She had to take charge of it. She imagined him waking, needing to escape because she'd discovered him. Her stomach had retched. She'd got out of the bath and vomited in the toilet bowl. She vomited him out of her. Her stomach would no longer be home to him. She never felt like that again.

"Compensation is really a distraction. It is the way professional misbehaviour is treated – made less serious for that," she said.

"No. Money doesn't sort it."

She said she wanted a public investigation. Compensation was only a side show, a distraction, a time waster, a way of avoiding reality.

Others spoke to the full room. One woman didn't mention her baby's death; it was too sacred to be mentioned there. She told of how she'd had a caesarean hysterectomy she didn't need. She said wanted a full inquiry into how all this happened.

Another woman was different; she almost wept for her baby. But she didn't. Instead she told how she watched her baby die for three days; she felt she would have been safer on the side of the road.

Yet another woman was just as wonderful. She spoke personally. She told of the lack of common humanity shown to her while in outpatients, how they suggested she was exaggerating her pain when she had a miscarriage. How her enormous loss was never acknowledged. How she feared her childbearing may have begun and ended that night too.

Then there came Cathriona. She was forthright and honest in her grief, describing how one of her ovaries was removed with her womb. She told of the lies that all the women were told: how they were bleeding to death, how they had placenta acretia; how none of it was true, according to pathology reports. How others in the hospital must have known; how a lot of others in the hospital had a lot of questions to answer too. It was not just Neary alone.

There was a stillness in the room while the women talked.

When Brendan McGahon spoke he annoyed the women and their husbands by suggesting we might be denying due process to Neary.

A woman stood up in the audience and confronted him. "Brendan, you're the very one who said rapists should be castrated."

"Are you saying Dr Neary should be castrated?" he asked.

"No, but something should be done about him and all the lies he told. All the women he mutilated. I shared an office with another of his victims. We thought it was something to do with electric static from the computers. How she believed he saved her life. And all along he was a madman."

Everyone supported her words.

I spoke for the first time, telling Brendan that he couldn't possibly understand what had happened after three hours. I had been listening to this story for three years and I hadn't fully come to terms with it. I told them that Dr John Bonnar was on record as saying that most obstetricians do two or three of these operations in their career and mostly on older women. Dr Neary did two on one night and performed two caesarean hysterectomies that I knew of on teenagers and two more on twenty-year-olds. Brendan seemed chastened after a woman in the audience reminded him of the lies they had all been told to cover up what was actually going on.

Seamus Kirk wanted it quantified.

"How can we quantify it?" Tony asked. "People have huge difficulty getting their own files, let alone quantifying it. That was for the politicians. Many files are missing. Why has nothing changed after the blood scandals? Why is it still the responsibility of the patient victim to rectify things?" he asked.

Colm, our solicitor, spoke of his proposal to set up a public inquiry and a compensation tribunal similar to the Stardust one. Twenty per cent of the files were missing or destroyed, he said. Some women were out of time. It would be cheaper in the long run.

Colm asked the politicians if they would sign his proposal. Most did.

Would they make representations to government about it? They promised they would. That they would be back to us in ten days.

In the end the women thought the meeting was very painful. However, it was necessary to tell their stories in order to bring some movement to what was a very slow and agonising struggle for them. In the long run, they wanted political support to improve care for others in the future. And they felt they got it.

Next morning Fergus O'Dowd, a Fine Gael county councillor from Drogheda called to say he was worried that the staff would not meet us. Tony had mentioned this. He asked me to phone the hospital manager, Declan Collins.

"Can I call you Sheila?" Declan asked when I called.

"Of course. It's my name."

Declan spoke of the letter I wrote to Mary Duff requesting a meeting, and told me it would be decided at the next management meeting at the end of the month. We never heard what this decision was.

I filled him in on the background and on my letter to Colette McCann. I felt it was very irresponsible to post copies of my letter to the Minister on the internet and then to send them to individual members of staff.

"It is on the record that it wasn't you who did it," he said.

On the Monday after our meeting with the politicians, RTÉ screened *No Tears*, a docudrama about the hepatitis C blood scandal. All that week when any of the women phoned, they said, "That's us on *No Tears*. Nothing has changed. That was us talking to the Minister. Except it was a different Minister. But maybe we will succeed like them and there will be a programme about us."

16

Brave Hearts

After the night in Drogheda, Nora Owen and Seamus Kirk, as the most senior local TDs, sought a meeting with Micheál Martin. As we waited for the outcome of this request to the Minister, a number of things happened.

News of our meeting broke in the papers after it arose at an NEHB meeting. The paper said that there was a call by Caoimhghín Ó Caoláin for a speeding-up of the Medical Council inquiry, a compensation tribunal and a full public inquiry. John Farrelly spoke about the harrowing experiences of the women and of the need to fast-forward the matter. Ó Caoláin's motion on asking the Medical Council to expedite matters was adopted by the NEHB.

At the end of January, Tony and I had an appointment with the Medical Council, the one rescheduled from July. This time I knew who people were: John Hillery, the vice-president of the Council, the psychiatrist who had attended the previous meeting, the Council registrar, Brian Lea; and

Dr Abdul Bulbulia. The blonde woman, Ger Feeney, turned up a little late. She is a nurse.

From the outset, the atmosphere was different. There was a little initial defensiveness on both sides, but it was acknowledged. Tony had an agenda prepared.

I warmed to John Hillery. He asked Tony and me how they could improve the knowledge the wider community had of their role. I told them that a former cabinet minister had mixed them up with the Irish Medical Organisation, so they needed a higher profile. They wondered how to approach journalists. The President of the Council, Professor Gerard Bury, joined us during the meeting, as did another lay member who had been held up in traffic. They invited us back at the end of March.

The first sign came that things were moving with the politicians. A letter from Nora Owen confirmed the request for a meeting with Minister Micheál Martin and all the local politicians for the following week.

I rang Minister Dermot Ahern's office to encourage him to turn up at the meeting with the Minister this time. I spoke to someone in his office again and reminded her of the Drogheda issue.

"The Minister was very sorry to miss the last meeting and he doesn't like to send a representative. He prefers to be there himself."

"That's great, because he has another opportunity to turn up next Wednesday. A meeting has just been arranged with the Minister for Health at 7.45 p.m. in his office. All the local representatives are invited."

"It's very short notice. The Minister is a very busy man."

"I know, but I only heard three minutes ago and it has just been arranged. This is the earliest possible notice."

"Oh." But she couldn't promise he would attend.

Deputy Seamus Kirk and I had a long and thoughtful conversation. He asked questions about background, numbers, distribution, comparisons with other areas. I told him of my involvement and how it came about. I told him of the missing records. Many women have no records, just a pathology report saying that their removed wombs were normal.

On 19 February, I was horrified by what I saw on the "Support Michael Neary" website. New allegations about other doctors at the hospital. Still the same stuff about me. I emailed the webmaster, saying it was defamatory and should be removed. Next day I got an email from them thanking me for my complaint and saying it had been removed.

On Wednesday, 27 February, the local TDs met Minister Micheál Martin at 9.45 p.m. in his office. After it, Deputy Seamus Kirk left a much-appreciated message on my mobile. Other TDs were keen to tell their constituents too. A large number of deputies had attended.

The meeting had been very brief. Micheál Martin had reiterated the results of the IOG's 1999 Report. He said the Medical Council needed four or five more meetings to conclude their investigation and the Minister's hands were tied until then. A further meeting with Patient Focus was offered. Seamus Kirk said the Council needed time because they had received about 200 complaints. This was the first I had heard of such numbers.

"They don't have to consider every case to decide if Neary is fit to be a doctor. A few would do, like in the Shipman case in Britain," I remarked.

"You see, the Medical Council is a law unto itself," he said.

"It can't be, Seamus. We are all answerable for our actions."

"If more cases got to court, it would help. How far on are the cases?" he asked.

"The second one is due before the courts in April." I had heard this from Allison Gough, whose case it was, in the previous few days.

"I see. Anyway, ask a delegation to meet the Minister."

"I'll do that."

The women didn't believe a decision was expected soon from the Medical Council. In October 2000 they had said they would be back in February 2001, then it would be June, then autumn, then March 2002. If Micheál Martin believed that, he would believe anything. That was only buying time. He had now become part of the problem.

I spoke to Noreen about Micheál Martin's new invitation to meet.

"Again," she said.

"Will you go?"

"I suppose we'll have to. It's better than not going. I have to do something about what Neary did to me."

Cathriona, however, was all against another visit to Micheál Martin. No more visits to politicians.

The Minister of State, Mary Wallace, offered a meeting and Nora Owen gave us good advice: "Make sure you accept the invitation from the Minister, otherwise you will look like the unreasonable ones. That's very important. Also, get a guarantee from him that he will keep tracks on the Medical Council."

Immediately after, I rang Seamus Kirk to ask him to set up the meeting.

By early March it was clear that the women were finding it difficult to appear on the RTÉ *Prime Time* television programme to talk about what had happened to them in Drogheda. They had met Mary Raftery and Sheila Ahern in early February in Drogheda. They liked and trusted them but it was still too painful to appear on a current affairs documentary.

"It would open me up too much again," one of the women said, speaking for most women at that time. "People would be looking at me and pointing me out again as the person something terrible had happened to. I wouldn't be able to look at it myself either, I don't think."

Teresa was going to do it, though. She had trusted Neary totally, prayed for him every night, lit candles in the local church on his behalf, in thanksgiving for her life. She had believed that she owed her very existence to him. However, the medical report on her operation was devastating in its honesty. She had needed neither the hysterectomy nor removal of ovaries. She would speak up for her daughters, for other women's daughters.

"We still need another woman to have a programme," the researcher said. I rang Noeleen, who told me she was still thinking about doing it.

Before being interviewed for the programme, I rang around the women to ask them what they wanted said. I felt

215

a huge responsibility to represent their feelings properly.

I talked to Nicola first. "Say he is cushioned by his profession. He is a free man. We live with the consequences."

Jenny said, "The Medical Council is not on our side. They are protecting him, hoping we will get tired, and he still swans round Monasterboice with the title 'doctor'. Nobody in the area will really believe us until he is stripped of that title. Until then, they won't believe. Patients are banging their heads off a brick wall dealing with the medical profession."

Linda talked about the teams of solicitors involved. "The legal system is very aggressive. Very sarcastic, very scathing. It is all very hurtful."

Niamh said, "I had nightmares about it last night even. I suppose I am suffering from post-traumatic stress. You know that thing. I wouldn't have coped without my family and the other women and the support I get from them."

Then there was the woman who told me, "I spend my life looking after other people's children to try and fill the hole."

And the girl who couldn't even do that yet because, as she said, "It underlines for me that I will never have any more."

My interview for *Prime Time* was in Sheila Ahern's large airy country kitchen in the Strawberry Beds. I arrived early, having left Aideen to school on my way. We had tea at her kitchen table. Two cockerels lived there, beautiful birds with combs on their heads and deep brown and white plumage, strutting their stuff.

"We keep hens too, in the back – they are separated from the cocks at the moment," Sheila said.

I wore my pink and white shirt and black trousers.

"Take your cardigan off when you're on telly," Aideen had said.

"Why?"

"It will look better. It's a bit sloppy," she added. "Trust me, I know about clothes."

"I'd better do as you say then." And I did.

When the producer Mary Raftery arrived, she got down to business quickly.

"This is a terrible story, but no one will talk. We have Teresa but we are relying on you today and Noeleen tomorrow. I hope she agrees. Otherwise I am not really sure we will have a programme. Why will nobody talk? Have they gone to counselling?"

"Yes, many of them have."

"No one in Drogheda will talk."

"It's just the stage of life most of them are at. A lot of them are very young. Younger women have things to do with their lives, careers to put together, relationships to nurture, children to rear. That's why it's mostly the older women who are talking. They have had more time to work things out."

"That's true," she said.

I was questioned for a couple of hours solid. I stopped in the middle for tea, which gave me more energy. But it was hard work. The cocks made so much noise as I told the story of my friends' lives that Sheila and Mary stopped the filming and let the cocks in with the hens. I was so absorbed that I never heard the cocks crow. Afterwards, when all was done, they filmed me at the computer in the study while Sheila rang Noeleen for her final decision. We all held our breaths, hoping desperately she would say yes. I got the thumbs up from Sheila: Noeleen had said yes. Andrew, Noeleen's son, would do it too. They had talked about it and decided.

"I hope she won't change her mind," Sheila said.

"Noeleen won't change her mind," I responded.

After her interview the next day, Noeleen rang to explain why she did it. "A sense of duty," she said. "I'm made like that. It's been a curse but there is nothing I can do about it. It runs in my family. My mother was the same. It took all day, from eleven o'clock," she went on. "I'm worn out. We even went downtown to film Andrew and me walking around. I decided to do that because you might as well be hung for a sheep as a lamb. I think Mary and Sheila were pleased with it. They said they were anyway, and they seemed happy."

Sheila rang later to say just how happy they were.

"You have a programme," I said.

"We sure have a programme. They were great. It was really powerful with the son next to his mother, standing up for her. Noeleen was great. Clear, and emotional too, when it was appropriate."

17

Hope Grows

On 14 March, Deirdre Gillane and I met in her office in the Department of Health and Children in Hawkins House. This had been arranged when we ran into each other at the making of a radio show about a week earlier.

"My office is a health hazard," she said as she offered me a cup of tea and a chair. I accepted both. She left for a few minutes and came back with the tea. The wallpaper on her computer was a skull and crossbones that constantly travelled across the computer face, disappeared for a moment and was then back again.

Deirdre's office was on the same floor as the Minister's. It was the standard principal officer's. She occupied a rectangular desk and a chair with its back to the window. We sat at a circular table in another corner. The office wasn't a health hazard. Its occupant worked hard. Several files were on the desk, but not dishevelled, merely waiting to be attended to.

I adopted the direct questioning strategy I had decided to use for future meetings. "What do you think happened in Drogheda, Deirdre?"

She was taken aback, but not alarmed. "It was terrible what happened there."

"How do you mean?"

"Well, it was horrendous."

"What was horrendous, Deirdre?"

"What he did."

"What did he do?"

"Well, he seemed to be doing his own thing."

"It was more than that, Deirdre. Dr Neary spoke a lot about blood, a lot about death to young women."

"I thought he was just an incompetent doctor."

"I don't believe that now. I did at the beginning but after three years things are different. You keep looking for explanations. You start off with the most benign and keep working up the line until you at last find one that fits the facts."

"Yes," she said.

I told her about the charges against Shine of sexually abusing boys. She had forgotten it. I told her Neary and Shine were part of a consortium who wanted to buy the Drogheda hospital at one point. I said it would all still be going on if the NEHB had not bought it instead.

She accepted that.

We talked about the Medical Council and how it was holding up everything; how it was impossible to get information from them.

"The Minister's hands are tied, that was his legal advice."

I said we accepted that the Minister was constrained but did not believe there was nothing he could do. After all, the

Council complained about the legislation they had to operate under and the Minister wasn't doing anything to help in a hurry.

"He could ask the Attorney General for his opinion," she suggested.

"I assumed he had done that by now."

"He could write to the Medical Council and ask to meet them about timescales. That was all they could talk about."

I accepted that.

Then she pointed to heads of a bill to reform the Medical Council sitting on her table. She offered me a copy for the women.

"The Minister had a very straight-talking meeting with the public representatives. A lot of them turned up and he wanted to set up a meeting with Patient Focus; 26 March at 7.00 p.m. was suggested." I agreed with this.

She spoke of the Valerie Neary case. "There was no liability there. And his own nurses went to him to have their babies," she said.

"I know, but she asked her husband on the way in not to let him remove her womb."

"I didn't know that," she said.

"She is very sick. That's why her case was fast-tracked through the system." She didn't know that either.

"The sooner more cases come up before the court the better," she said.

"There's another soon. After Easter," I told her.

Our fourth meeting with the Minister took place on 26 March 2002. Tony, Colm, Celia, Patrick, Noeleen, Maura and Pat, and myself represented Patient Focus; Deirdre

Gillane accompanied the Minister. Mary Wallace, Seymour Crawford, Rory O'Hanlon, Senator Ann Leonard (who, it turned out, had been a nurse at Our Lady of Lourdes) and Caoimhghín Ó Caoláin also attended. The last two stayed throughout the meeting, which lasted about two hours.

Colm outlined the legal position and what Patient Focus wanted regarding tribunals of inquiry and of compensation. He pointed out the legal difficulties surrounding the Statute of Limitation, the trauma of patients, lack of files, which were missing, lost, destroyed or perhaps removed conveniently.

"The advantage of a redress board is it would save money," Colm said.

The last point did not appeal to Micheál Martin. "The legal profession will always find ways of making money. People could get money for jam with a set-up like that. Trauma is the most important reason as to why a redress scheme is needed," the Minister said.

"The onus of proof needs to be changed for the lost files," Colm said. "A lot of files are missing. It should be up to the defendant to prove there was no negligence in this case."

"I have pressed the Medical Council for information about progress in the investigation and they told Deirdre after several requests that they hoped it would be available in two months," the Minister told the meeting.

"Do you believe them?"

He thought for a moment. "I don't believe anything any more. I am precluded from interfering with them," he added once again.

Afterwards Colm said he felt a weight off his shoulders. The women would get what they needed in the end.

Teresa's Story

Michael Neary removed Teresa's womb after she had her baby in 1992. He removed her ovaries too. She looks very young and trim to have four children and looks more like a sister to her lovely daughters than a mother. She has a son too; her last baby.

"I found it very hard to cope with my baby afterwards," she told me the first time we spoke. *"I was very depressed and crying a lot. Dr Neary told me I was bleeding to death and that he had saved my life. I was just turned forty. He removed my ovaries as well as my womb. He said I had endometriosis. I had to get on with my life. I was due to attend Dr Neary the day the news about his practice broke. I rang the hospital. They told me to attend anyway. I saw another doctor but she couldn't answer any of my questions about my operation. But she got my files for me. I appreciated that. I didn't receive any blood, so I was not bleeding to death anyway. Maybe I had endometriosis,"* she said.

Now she says, "I totally believed Dr Neary saved my life. I prayed for him and lit candles at the church for him all the time. I thanked God for him every night. He was like a father in the theatre. Very tender really. I put my hands round his neck as he helped me on to the operating table in the theatre that day, I trusted him so much. Dr Porter told me I didn't need a hysterectomy and neither did I need my ovaries removed. I feel very upset now. I have gone from totally being grateful to him to knowing he assaulted me. I feel gutted that the guards are not going to follow up on the complaint I made to them. I am really cross about that."

Many of the women tell the self-same story.

18

Broken Trust

The trailer for *Broken Trust,* the *Prime Time* documentary, gave me a physical shock. Presenter Miriam O'Callaghan's voice spoke of "one doctor, one hospital, dozens of young women stripped of their wombs in childbirth, for no apparent reason". The picture of the theatre, the masked gowned man, the surgical instruments, the male voice saying that some aspects of this story were so extraordinary they almost beggared belief. This was Dr Richard Porter, one of the doctors the women had consulted. I was physically afraid listening to him. He gave weight to what I knew.

I saw it first after the Sunday news. Noeleen and Teresa were so quietly spoken yet so definite. Teresa asked if Neary had just targeted naïve women. Noeleen said she had never heard of women having a hysterectomy when having a baby until it happened to her.

Wilfie and I poured a glass of red wine and sipped some during the programme. Before the showing Teresa and Noeleen had both phoned, scared of how they would be seen and treated after going public. I suggested wine for them too. It helped me sit through the programme. As the credits rolled, the phone tolled. First was Cathriona, then Tony, Emily, Colm and Jenny. Then Jim Reilly phoned. He and Declan Collins were manning the helpline. I was on the phone until midnight. I didn't sleep for hours.

The next day was chaotic. Six new women came forward, the first time I had spoken to so many new people in one day. It was more of the same old familiar story, but each woman's voice was different, each had a different emphasis. One described how she was one of "the lucky ones". Neary didn't remove her womb.

I cried several times that day. Once was when I heard Sara on *Loose Talk* on LMFM. She spoke of her terrible year after her baby was born and her womb was removed. She talked of depression and family problems. She spoke of the terrible loneliness of never having another child. Never a day goes by for her without several reminders, such as friends or sisters-in-law having babies. Each time her son reaches a milestone she knows she will never see that again. All the women said that. Birthdays are also anniversaries; babygros are folded away with grief; first steps are also the only first steps; first days at school are bereavements. There is a clinging onto the milestones.

We needed more doctors to help. Tony would sort that, as ever.

Mary Raftery and Sheila Ahern both rang to see if the women liked the programme. Mary Raftery also checked if a young woman who rang her had got in touch. Both her ovaries had been removed by Neary.

"The women loved the programme and, yes, she did make contact."

I got two nuisance calls also.

Later that week I got a phone call from Marie Kierans of the *Drogheda Independent*. She wanted to talk to one of the women for a piece in the following Wednesday's paper. She wanted to know if I understood that there was a lot of support for the doctor in the town. "Not being local, you wouldn't know that," she said.

"The Bristol baby doctors were heavily supported too. That means nothing." She'd had her babies in Drogheda, she said.

I explained that most of the women affected were not from Drogheda and that might influence the way the town looked at matters. Maybe some hadn't come forward because of the attitude in the town. She asked where I was from and how I got involved. I told her of course. "I am just the co-ordinator. Most of the work now is done by local women." I told her she must be nice to the women if they spoke to her. I promised I would pass on her number to a few. But the women would decide.

I phoned Noeleen. Andrew answered the phone. He was very pleased he had done the programme. "About ten people came up to me today and congratulated me and sympathised with me." He would ask his mother about talking to the paper. She was out. "People are taking it on board now that this was really bad and it went on for twenty years. You don't get Brownie points when you save someone that gives you the right to damage someone else," he said. "I can't understand that logic."

I phoned Nicola. "The paper was unfair to the women," she said. "There was front-page reporting of the march in support of Neary and of the applause he got when he arrived in a pub in Drogheda after it. Then, when he was suspended, there was just a little notice in the inside. No headlines this time. No, I don't think I'll talk to her. Even last week's editorial was supporting him. I can't stand the name Drogheda now. I hate going there. I wish I could pick Drogheda up and throw it into the sea," she said.

We were laughing again. Nicola always laughs.

I rang Sara. After being on the radio, she might be ready for another outing.

"I am really glad I did it. A midwife at the hospital called to the house last night with a box of chocolates. They were all listening to it at the hospital. My husband couldn't believe I did it. I just got so angry at people ringing up saying we were doing it for money. I couldn't help myself." I left Marie Kierans' number with Sara.

I passed on Nicola's message to Marie Kierans. Hospitals weren't about business and politics. They were about patients. "The women think that your paper thinks it's about business. Some don't really want to talk to you. Others might." Her attitude softened.

"I will read back to them what I write," she said.

A very short time later, Darren Hughes rang. "I'm the group editor for the *Drogheda Independent* and the Fingal local paper." He explained that he was only in the job three months and that things were changing. He worked on the radio station and he was well briefed on the situation. He had been speaking to Marie Kierans and he specifically apologised for the previous week's editorial. In effect, he said it was written by the lawyers ten minutes before it was due to be printed. He would email me an apology.

"We're afraid of being sued by lots of consultants in the hospital, any consultant who ever passed through it," he admitted. That explained a lot.

"Thank you for that. I appreciate it and I'll pass it on to the women."

Part 4

Public Acknowledgement

19

Allison's Case

On a beautiful spring day in April 2002 Allison Gough's civil case against Michael Neary opened in the High Court. I had spent the previous two days in the Four Courts as she waited for a judge, while her legal team were in talks with Neary's team. I knew Allison had been longing for this day – her day in court. I had seen her only once at our meetings but Fergus, her husband, always came and she often phoned. Her solicitor had advised her that it would be wiser not to attend our meetings as it could be said it would affect her story if she heard others.

I knew that Allison had a clear mind, a strong sense of morality, and a profound need for justice. She needed vindication for herself, for her family, for the other women. There was a need to expose the truth in open court, a need to feed and water it with her words and to see it bloom and multiply by means of a judge's unbiased decision. I knew she would not easily settle, that it would take a lot to persuade her. In fact, I believed nothing could persuade her. She reminded me of the bluebells in our garden. Katie planted one in a yoghurt pot when she was in fourth class. It was my Mother's Day gift that year. She is twenty-one now and her bluebell turned into hundreds when transferred to open ground and exposed to the sun. Allison needed to tell what Neary did in open court, expose it to the sun. Other women would grow strength from her truth.

There was the hustle and bustle of the marketplace in Court Number 1 as people gathered for the opening of the case. Men in black came and went, whispering about placentas, caesarean hysterectomies, bleeding. I saw Professor John Bonnar take a seat in front. The hospital staff (all women, mostly midwives, I am told) are all together in the back row behind me. They have a lot of documents on their laps. Allison and her husband are over to the left.

Allison wept through her testimony. She gave simple answers to direct questions. She had been Dr Lynch's patient but was admitted to be induced on the October bank holiday weekend in 1992. Dr Neary was on duty when midwives rang him and said that her baby was in distress and needed to be delivered. She was twenty-seven years of age. She was nervous, having her first baby. She said she had a difficult time. She told of how when she woke after the caesarean section, the nurse told her she had a baby boy and that he was fine.

She described how she was told her womb was gone. The day after the birth of her baby, Dr Neary walked by her bed. She told him she could not sleep after the birth.

"If you did not sleep, how do you think I felt?" was his reply.

Next day he came again and she asked if she could have a section if she had more babies. He said, "What do you mean, more babies? I had to do a hysterectomy."

Allison said that she broke down then.

"I saved your life," he said.

"He then said he could have sent my son home without a mammy. That I lost so much blood, he never saw anything like it. Then he left. For two years of my son's life I felt no joy. I was just there in body."

She said that she was afraid they would take her baby off her if she told them this. She blamed herself.

"At the six-weeks check up I asked Dr Neary if I did anything wrong. I asked him to explain what happened to me, why I lost my womb. He said if he told me what happened that night I would never sleep again. He told me to go home and get on with my life.

"I feel guilty now I didn't ask more questions. Maybe I could have saved some of the women. I was one of the first, you see." I believe if she had been able to attend the meetings she would have been less hard on herself about this.

Fergus looked on from the side as his wife bore witness. She spoke directly to the judge.

Allison and Fergus were heartbroken as Professor John Bonnar gave his testimony. He told how only one woman in 100,000 would be expected to have a hysterectomy giving birth for the first time, and then only for massive bleeding or cancer. Allison had neither. More should have been done to conserve her womb. There was too quick a rush to remove it. Neary's barrister repeatedly suggested that Allison could have died.

"Mrs Gough would have died if she was giving birth in Jenin Refugee Camp. But she was in an Irish hospital, wasn't she?" Justice Johnson said.

Dr Mary Wingfield told of how devastated Allison was when she came to see her. She had not had a massive bleed.

From 1990 to 1998 there hadn't been a single caesarean hysterectomy in the National Maternity Hospital in a first-time mother, Dr Wingfield told the court.

Two Irish obstetricians had spoken up for Allison! Everyone had said that Irish doctors would not speak against each other. Well, the much-respected John Bonnar did. So too did the young, soft-spoken and very professional Dr Mary Wingfield. *It's good that Allison has a woman doctor speaking for her*, I thought.

Allison's psychiatrist, Dr McCarthy, said she needed justice and the court process to recover. He spoke about Allison's need to tell her story. Dr Neary had told her he had saved her life and people said she should send him a thank you card. Dr McCarthy spoke of how important the much-derided legal process is for Allison's recovery.

Next it was the turn of the defendant; it was Michael Neary's turn to give evidence.

About twenty or so of the women turned up to hear Neary give evidence. They came together, they came with their husbands, with their mothers, with their friends. The midwives from the hospital consulted their documents. The day before, Allison had called me to make sure no one would shout at him. I had got on the phone to deliver Allison's message. Everyone had to be quiet.

"He will probably lie through his teeth, but you have to sit still and listen for Allison, for everyone," was what I told them.

The atmosphere had been very tense before Neary actually came into the court room. Justice Johnson had just delivered his decision on the first question argued by Neary's defence team, that it had been too long ago to take a case. The judge ruled that Allison did not have knowledge that she may have been damaged by Neary until the news about him broke just before Christmas in 1998. She had gone to her solicitor immediately on hearing this news. So she was not debarred.

Neary took the witness box in his own defence. This large, silver-haired man was dressed in a dark grey suit, blue shirt and yellow tie. He carried a large brown soft leather bag that he placed on the floor and would fumble in for documents during his questioning. A garda stood at each door with his arrival. Neary seemed a little nervous as he answered the easy questions about his name and qualifications at the start of his evidence. But he settled in, and very quickly became confident and unflappable.

He qualified as a doctor in 1965 from University College Galway, he said. He qualified as an obstetrician in 1970. He spent two years as an intern in Galway, then he went to England as a Senior House Officer and Registrar in Obstetrics. He told how there were three obstetricians in the Lourdes, Dr O'Brien, Dr Lynch and himself. Dr O'Brien was off sick. As a rule, he would not consult with Dr Lynch in difficult cases, because Dr Lynch was his junior. He hadn't read the report of the Institute of Obstetricians and Gynaecologists in four years, so he was not familiar with its findings about his practice of caesarean hysterectomy at the Lourdes.

He remembered Allison's delivery on 26 October 1992 very well. It was about the time that the hepatitis C scandal broke and there was anxiety about giving blood to women. He had saved her life, he said; if she had not had a hysterectomy, she would have bled to death. It took thirty to forty minutes to do the hysterectomy.

"One would massage the womb all the time once the bleeding started until the hysterectomy started," he said. He had manipulated her womb and packed it with hot packs, but had not recorded this because it was his routine. He did do it, he said; he always did it. "One doesn't record routine," he told the judge.

Also, he testified that he didn't alter the records afterwards to make things look better for himself. "I wouldn't do that. It would be unethical." He wrote his operation notes in red pen, he said.

He knew a hysterectomy would be a very upsetting and traumatic event for a young woman having her first baby. "I went over the night of Allison's operation a thousand times in my head."

He said too that it was not in his character to say to a woman that she would never sleep again if she knew what had happened in theatre, or that her son could have gone home without a mammy if it were not for him. She would be distressed and confused after the surgery, as is normal in any woman. To say these things would induce fear in the patient. It would be outrageous to say to a patient, "If you knew what happened last night in theatre you would never sleep again". All this he told the judge and the full court of women, who knew he said it or things like it many times.

"Are you afraid to look at what you did that night because if you did you could not live with yourself afterwards?" Allison's barrister asked Neary.

After a pause he replied, "No."

Of the ten hospital staff in the theatre that night only Neary gave evidence. The midwives who attended court were getting greyer and more tired as each day went by. As Neary gave his evidence, they consulted documents.

The women looked and listened. There was no shouting, no abuse, only silence in the public gallery for Neary's evidence. An elderly doctor was called for the defence case too. His evidence was that he could not say if the hysterectomy was needed or not unless he had been in the theatre when Allison had her baby. The case was then adjourned.

"Neary was like a clown in the witness box," Allison told me on the phone some days after the hearing of evidence was over. "Last night was the first night in ages I slept. I can't believe the reaction of people in Ardee. I am getting cards and flowers from complete strangers." At a school function the local sergeant had come up and shaken her hand.

"I'd recommend all the women to do what I am doing," she said. "I have lost a stone since this started because I can't eat but it's well worth it. When this is over I am not giving any interviews. I am going to concentrate on Fergus and my son. I will be there for the women, but I need to put my life back together."

I think Allison had planted the flower of truth in fertile soil. I believed in time it would multiply.

Every night after the hearings my phone rang constantly, many calls from women who could not get to court asking for news, but also some from new women. I was disturbed by some young women who told me he had removed their ovaries but did not remove their womb. They were in their twenties and early thirties.

Tony and I had our second follow-up meeting with the Medical Council in late April. Tony prepared a paper outlining our concerns and sent it to the Council. Among the issues raised was the question of delay in relation to correspondence from patients.

John Hillery chaired the meeting. Also there was Abdul Bulbulia, Brian Lea, a lay woman council member, Tony and me. Ger Feeney and Gerard Bury joined later. They went on the offensive immediately after polite chit-chat. They asked: Who are you? We can't find you in any phone book. Who are your committee? Who funds you? What is your relationship with the Department of Health? To whom are you accountable? I was surprised they had waited until now to ask questions like this.

Tony replied to these queries. I told them how some women with complaints about Dr Neary had never received a reply to their letters.

"All correspondence is acknowledged within a reasonable time."

"What do you mean by reasonable? Is it six weeks, six months, a year?"

"Everything is acknowledged within six weeks," I was firmly told.

"Some of the women in the Neary group never got an acknowledgement of their complaints. They were sent to the Council in late January 1999 and they have yet to receive a reply of any sort. Others too."

I was asked for their names and addresses, in writing. I offered to give them there and then – their names at any rate; I was very familiar with them.

"It would waste the time of the meeting if you were to tell us now," they said.

"All I expect is that you believe this and ensure it doesn't happen again. I don't want to make a big to do about it. I don't want to turn into you," I added. Understandably, John Hillery was very offended. I corrected myself. "I don't mean you personally; I mean the Medical Council."

He wanted to end the meeting. He stood up. Heads were nodding in disapproval all around the table. I felt the cold wind of social ostracism.

Abdul Bulbulia changed the subject and went through Tony's submission. He said he agreed with seventy-five to eighty per cent of it.

"We don't want to destroy the Council. Just improve it," Tony said.

Most of their comments were addressed to Tony now. They talked of how they had difficulty with the legislative framework of the Council. They wished it changed but were not having much luck politically. It was not a priority for government. Tony could help with this. He could put pressure on the Minister.

Abdul said that Tony's skills were useful and suggested that there might be other skilled people in our organisation who could contribute. They invited us back again in September to further the discussions. That was the last straw for me.

"I understand that you prefer to talk to Tony because he is a doctor and you are more comfortable with him. However, I speak to ordinary people every day whose views matter. I am trying to represent their views honestly. And I am not totally unskilled academically." I heard myself list my academic qualifications. I have never had to do this in my life before. I like to think I can acquit myself reasonably in most company.

The whole attitude to me changed with these simple comments. The scowls were gone, eye contact established again. Suddenly I was in the room. Abdul even suggested I contribute to the forthcoming revision of the ethical guidelines.

"I would be happy to," I said.

After, I said to Tony, "I don't know why I bother."

"Because it matters," he said.

I sent details of the six women's lack of acknowledgement to their complaints in the afternoon post in two separate letters, each with details of three women in no particular combination. Nicola and Noreen were two of the women involved in one letter, along with another woman, as not having received acknowledgements.

Ever since the *Prime Time* programme had gone out I had been feeling very uneasy. Between it and Allison's case, a large number of new women were getting in touch. My phone was ringing all the time. There were now over eighty women in the group. Each new woman in the main told the same old story: how Neary removed her womb while she was having a baby; how he told them he saved their life; the same trauma, the same disbelief. I never got used to it. Each time I thought it would end all right. I reassured them all that they may have needed the surgery. After all, Neary didn't injure everyone. We would refer them to a doctor who would provide them with an independent report, which would be paid for by the health board. They should take it one step at a time.

I had a feeling that the worst cases were coming out now because of a new trend: women whose ovaries were removed in their twenties and early thirties who were told they were pre-cancerous or that they had a condition called endometriosis. Perhaps Teresa's story on *Prime Time* sparked these women to contact us, or perhaps it was what Dr Richard Porter had said about her, especially about the removal of her ovaries at forty. If she was his wife, he said, and this happened to her, he would be incandescent. I was becoming disturbed. Was there a lot more to this story than we knew? Were three or four cases of young women whose ovaries were removed enough to establish a trend?

It was Sinead's phone call that solidified these feelings. She was one of the new women. She had got her notes from the hospital and had been looking at them. The fact that her pathology report said her cysts were benign and that the word "benign" was underlined alarmed her. Neary had told her they were pre-cancerous. It alarmed me too. What was going on? Why were her ovaries removed then? She was a young married woman who wanted children. She was not sick. The ovaries had no complicating factor like supposed blood loss, as in the caesarean hysterectomies. This was frightening me.

"He said I was just the third person this ever happened to," Sinead continued. "He said that he left my operation and got advice. I wanted to talk to one of the others but Neary later told me he had consulted them and they didn't want to talk to me."

Sinead sought a medical opinion which confirmed that she did not need the surgery. The doctor apologised to her for what had happened – that a member of his profession had done this to her.

I was looking forward to meeting Sinead and the other recent callers at a meeting in the Boyne Valley. About fifteen of them came. Noeleen and Teresa helped to settle their fears. The two young women who had had both ovaries removed were there. This was chilling my bones; Tony's too. The atmosphere was shy at first but in the end we stayed talking until midnight. The talk too was of awaiting judgment day at the High Court.

Two letters arrived from the Medical Council, one during May, the other in July. In the first they said they were writing to Nicola and Noreen to apologise for not keeping them informed of what was going on in relation to their case and for not acknowledging their original letters of complaint. They said they never received the third letter of complaint. I accepted this.

The July letter was similar and concerned the other three women who had not received acknowledgements. One of the women named in the second letter was May. The Council would write to two named women to apologise about the lack of communication. But there was no record of any written complaint from May. I couldn't believe it. I had personally placed May's letter in with Nicola's and Noreen's in one envelope when the women complained to the Medical Council after our first meeting in January 1999. If they had received Nicola's and Noreen's, they must have received hers.

I rang the Council registrar, who agreed to look into that case again. I told him he must look for the letters. The women were telling the truth. I reckoned they had both these missing letters, but knew for sure they had one. The registrar promised to get back to me.

Some days later he called. "I don't know if this is good or bad news, but we found one of the missing letters, May's. A fax of it turned up in our solicitor's office."

"That's definitely good. But what about the other woman? I totally believe her. She knows what she is talking about."

"There was a meeting of the full Council yesterday and it arose. We are going to do an audit of our system with a third party overseeing it."

"Good. Because this is awful."

"Everyone can make a mistake," he said.

"Yes, of course. But institutions seem to have difficulty admitting them."

"Well, I know they do. But letters don't get 'lost', only 'mislaid', so we will be writing to both women," he said.

"When you're writing to the woman whose letter was mislaid, make sure you ask her if she wants to continue with the complaint. She is a quiet woman and may well feel the exercise of complaining to the Medical Council is a waste of time at this stage."

"Oh, we will, of course."

I was reassured that the Registrar understood the seriousness of what had happened.

I rang Tony. He would find out who the "independent auditor" was. I was so pleased I couldn't stop smiling. I rang Nicola and told her about the smile on my face.

In October, when I returned from holidays, a letter from the Medical Council, with its now familiar logo, was waiting. It was from John Hillery. The tone was warm and encouraging, beginning "Dear Ms O Connor" which was crossed out in handwriting and replaced with "Dear Sheila", and ending with "Yours sincerely, John". The review of procedures was underway. He thanked me for the letters, saying they had been very important, and he requested the women's permission to pass them on to the review.

20

Meeting Kathryn

The first time I met Kathryn Quilty was in late October in Ardee, in the hospital outside the town. It was a large red-bricked building with very few cars in the car park on a Saturday afternoon. Ardee is a psychiatric hospital.

I had been wondering about this girl since the very beginning. I knew there were four young women who had been nineteen or twenty when Neary removed their wombs. So far, only two of them were in our group. So when Kathryn's solicitors emailed Tony, I was very pleased. I phoned them immediately.

The solicitors, Michael Boylan and Gillian O'Connor, came to my house the following week. "The scandal is that this isn't a scandal," Gillian said.

They wanted to have a look at me before they asked me to contact Kathryn. I liked this very protective approach. Kathryn had been in Ardee a week by then, they said.

Helen, Niamh's mother, came with me. She brought Kathryn a lovely gift, a very girly handbag of toiletries. The door of Unit 1 was locked. We tried the door a few times before anyone came to let us in. A strong young man unlocked the door at last. His body blocked the entrance. He said nothing.

"We're looking for Kathryn Quilty. I think she is in Unit One," I said. A nurse came by and looked at us. "Kathryn Quilty?" I said again.

"She's in there," the nurse said. The strong man moved away from the doorway to allow us into the small hall, locked the door behind us and disappeared. The still hovering nurse repeated, "She's in there."

She pointed past the TV room, with games of Scrabble, Monopoly and cards on tables, into a ward with about fifteen or twenty beds. It was hard to see where one room ended and another began. Old-style hospital blankets – the pale blue ones with the open crochet in them – covered each bed. Some beds were empty. A nurse sat by one holding a young woman's hand. Tenderness in a bleak building.

A frail, pale, young girl looked up from another bed. She walked towards us. She was dressed in a light blue jumper and blue jeans, with a pleat from the knees down and lined with white cotton lace. She was very thin, about six and a half stone and five foot three. She had long blonde hair, like Niamh's.

"Kathryn?" I asked.

"Yes?"

"I'm Sheila and this is Helen, Niamh's mother."

"Was Niamh a patient of Neary's too?"

"Yes," Helen said. "And she was young, like you."

"I didn't know there were others," she said to Helen. "We can talk privately over here." Kathryn was pointing in the direction we had come in.

We walked in through the TV room, through the small hall into a hallway-type room with several tables surrounded by chairs. It was very open but Kathryn ushered us to sit down.

"Thanks for coming," she said. "Since this happened I have felt all alone – me and my little boy. I feel very bad that I'm not with him now. But I couldn't cope; I tried to cope, but I can't eat or get up. People say I am always frowning. I never smile. I can't remember when I laughed. I never was like that. I was happy and contented. I had another operation in September because I have other problems after my hysterectomy, so I can't hold my son."

A nurse called over to us, "No smoking, ladies."

Kathryn got up. "Come on, we'll go to the smoking room." The smoking room was filthy – cold, hard, metal chairs. Brown floors and walls, window wide open. There was another patient, a man, there too. It was difficult to talk. But we did anyway.

"I don't feel like a woman any more," Kathryn said. Helen and Kathryn talked as much as was possible. When they finished their cigarettes, we went back into the ward to Kathryn's bed. "They want me to go home for the day tomorrow but I don't want to go. I don't like going out."

Kathryn didn't know about our group. We told her we would invite her to all our meetings, that she should bring her mother and/or her partner. I told her I would ring her every week. "It's tender loving care the women in our group give; that's what you'll get from them."

She smiled quietly but I thought she was pleased. There was a little bit of comfort in her face, as if she could imagine the love of the women and thought she wanted it. Helen reassured her.

Kathryn showed us pictures of her little boy.

"He's very happy always smiling" she said. They send me pictures of him from Baldoyle. It's very nice of them. He is happy there but he must be home for Christmas."

There were painted bottles on the windowsill behind Kathryn's bed. One was red and glittered; very Christmassy. The other was of the sky, a daisy touching it, and a field. I thought them very beautiful.

The last thing she said before we left was that she was looking forward to meeting Niamh. That was the important connection. Helen was the mother of a girl like her. Later, on the way home in the car, I said this to Helen. Then we talked about Kathryn's beautiful bottles.

"I didn't go home on Sunday," Kathryn told me when I phoned the following Thursday, Hallowe'en.

"Oh, that's a pity; what happened?"

"I couldn't. I was terrified of going out. I just wanted to curl up under the duvet. But I'm going home for the weekend this week and I am expected to be going home for good the week after."

"Oh, that's great news."

"Is there any news about the meetings?" she asked.

"No. There's no news of Allison's case yet. Don't worry, I won't forget you?"

"What's the case?"

"It's the first case to be fully heard in the High Court," I told her. "We are just waiting for a judgment. We're hoping for it any day now."

"When will it be?"

"Not sure, but very soon, we expect. In November anyway. We will arrange a meeting then. The women and their families will have to decide what to do. I hope you'll come yourself and your mother and partner too."

"Yeah, I'm looking forward to that. I always thought I was alone."

"No, you're not alone, Kathryn. How are you?"

"A bit better," she said.

"Good. You have a lot to look forward to, Kathryn. You and your little boy."

"I know," she said.

We said goodbye.

I felt happier.

Following the 2002 General Election, Fine Gael had a new spokesperson on Health, Olivia Mitchell. Tony and I met with her on 12 November. Tony was delayed, and Olivia appeared rushed as she took my name and our phone numbers. I decided to get down to business immediately.

"I am involved with an organisation called Patient Focus. We are a patient advocacy group; we deal with difficulties people have with the health care system, usually hospitals and consultants. We are dealing with the Neary case."

But Olivia did not know of the Neary scandal. We had spent the last three years going around the TDs in Dáil Éireann. We'd talked to John Bruton, Michael Noonan, Gay Mitchell. They had never told her, or if they did, she did not remember. So many people hadn't heard, despite all our work. I was very grateful to Olivia for her lack of pretence. We needed to know the message was not really getting out.

"We're sick going to see Micheál Martin. He seems to think that all he has to do is grant people an audience and there's the case solved," I said. She was listening carefully. "We haven't brought the women with us this time because honestly it would be an insult to ask them to tell their stories again," I explained.

Olivia was looking straight at me, leaning back on her chair. Calm. She had stopped taking notes.

"Is he still practising?"

I told her about the Medical Council and that by now about eighty women were involved with Patient Focus, and many were taking legal action. Then I told her about Shine. About Drogheda, about the others who must have known.

"What do ye want?" she asked. "A medical ombudsman?"

"Yes, of course, but that won't happen for another five years or so."

"It could happen tomorrow." The division bells started to ring in the background. She said nothing, just kept looking at me.

"There's the division bells, do you have to go?"

"Yes, but I'll be back."

She was away about five minutes. Tony was just arriving by then. I was glad to see him. He spoke to Olivia about medical litigation and how we could prevent it. She seemed at sea. She had no idea about all this but was very keen to help.

"Have you funding? Maybe I can help there."

"The NEHB are funding us a little," Tony said.

By now it was 5.25. She had to go.

"I'll have to get legal advice on this."

"You could ask a parliamentary question about the Medical Council and its delaying."

"He will just say it is not for him."

"No, he has answered before and quite fully. Talk to Liz McManus," I said.

"I don't want to do any harm." This was absolutely genuine.

"You won't, Olivia, you won't. But do something."

Next morning while I was thinking about the meeting with Olivia, and feeling totally fed up, the phone rang. It was Allison. She had a date. "It's Friday at 11.00," she said.

"The judgment?"

"Yeah."

"I'll be there."

"You can tell everyone."

"I'll get on the blower and tell as many as I can," I said.

I spent that afternoon on the phone, spreading the news through our contact network. Women I called rang other women.

In the post that day there was another letter from the Medical Council's John Hillery. This time I am "Dear Sheila"; no need to cross out the typed "Dear Ms O Connor" this time. *"The review will be carried out by Senior Counsel."* It listed the terms of reference. *"The Senior Counsel concerned is I believe Mr Harry Whelehan. He has been asked to report to the Council at the earliest possible date."* It was signed "John".

I told some of the women. We were being taken seriously at last.

Fidelma's Story

Fidelma Geraghty is striking for her competence and assurance, a woman in her mid-thirties who is used to managing a team in IBM, having people do as she asks. She is from The Naul, a rural area in North Dublin. She makes decisions with assurance and sticks by them. She is warm and funny too, a lovely person to have a meal with. You can absolutely depend on Fidelma. She carries her abilities and achievements lightly. She is the sort of woman we all want to be and would like our daughters to become.

It is difficult to imagine her as victim, let alone a victim of Michael Neary's. And yet she was for a while, until she was instrumental in ensuring his reign of terror in Our Lady of Lourdes Hospital was made public.

She is married to Vincent and has two girls, Ellen and Jenny. But Fidelma and Vincent had another baby and Ellen and Jenny another sister. Baby Hannah was delivered by Neary on 1 October 1997. Fidelma knew their third child would be born dead, because scans showed that Hannah suffered from a rare condition, which meant she would not survive.

Fidelma had been attending Neary since hearing this terrible news about ten weeks earlier after scans in the Rotunda following a car accident. He had delivered Ellen and Jenny, so it was natural she would attend him. When I visit their home and sit in their large beautiful front room I see pictures of baby Hannah's little feet and hands side by side with those of two other gorgeous babies. Little baby Hannah is a much-loved and remembered family member.

When Fidelma went into hospital for a prearranged section to deliver Hannah, she knew it would be painful and grief-ridden, but she did not expect any more. A recent scan had shown the baby's heartbeat could not be found. Neary was very kind and compassionate to her. Everything was to happen when she was ready, it was agreed.

She delivered Hannah under epidural, so she was awake for her baby's birth. Her husband Vincent was with her. But during the section Neary told her she was bleeding very heavily; she could die, he told her, if he did not intervene swiftly. What he had to do was to remove her womb.

The atmosphere in theatre was calm and businesslike. Vincent did not see a lot of blood. But Fidelma totally trusted her doctor. After all, why wouldn't she?

"You're a mess inside. I have to remove everything," Neary told her as soon as little Hannah was delivered. He could not save her ovaries, he said, because one of them was gangrenous and the placenta was interwoven with her womb and second ovary. He held the removed ovary and womb up for her to see. She felt it was unreal, looking on at a piece of

tissue just cut from her, but she believed it was to save her life.

Later Neary told Vincent he was lucky not to be taking his wife home in a box. They believed it. Of course they did.

They tried to get on with life because they had two beautiful girls to bring up. Now they knew they would not have the large family they planned for, but they had a lot to be happy about. And that is what they did. And they were very grateful to the doctor who saved Fidelma so she could return to her family.

Over the following years she heard the news of his suspension from the Medical Register and the investigation into his practice, but she never thought it applied to her. He had been charming and considerate to her. He had saved her life. Her story was different. She did not think otherwise, not even for a second. Not until she saw The Late Late Show, that is, and heard Maria, Noeleen and the other women in the audience tell their stories. They were describing her experience word for word. She knew there and then that she too was one of Neary's victims.

Fidelma learned later that her files were missing. Only a photocopy of some of her hospital notes were ever found. They turned up in a search of Neary's home after it was raided by the gardaí some years later. It mattered terribly that at least this small amount of notes were discovered. Otherwise she could not have grieved properly for the babies she and Vincent did not have, for the brothers or sisters denied to Ellen and Jenny, for the grandchildren denied to her and Vincent's parents. She at least had some answers, unlike the other forty-three women whose files were never found.

255

She found out then that she had not been bleeding to death; in fact, the blood that had been ready for her was sent back to the laboratory. She also learned that another young mother had had her womb removed on that 1 October by Neary. She didn't hear this during her stay in the hospital; she learned of it from the judge who inquired into the whole affair.

(As told to me and Cathriona and as told to Suzanne Power and published in the Sunday Tribune *Features magazine, 31 August 2008.)*

21

The High Court Finds for Allison

It was pouring rain and had been for the last thirty-six hours. The rain and wind was torrential in the north-east. The previous night Allison was in excited mood but now the weather had halted everything. The roads in from Ardee and Kells were flooded. The women rang; some were on their way, some were stranded.

The women who lived nearest could come. Cathriona couldn't. She was mad with herself. Nicola couldn't either. I would ring them as soon as there was news. Tony arrived. Wilfie was with me that day. I headed into the Four Courts again.

The handing down of the judgment in Court Number 1 happened in a flash.

"Judgment with costs to the plaintiff, Mrs Gough."

I had to do a double take. "What did he say?" Wilfie repeated it. Did I hear right? €273,000 in damages? Copies of the judgment were handed out.

Leave to appeal was requested. "Wait until you read the judgment first," Judge Johnson said to Neary's barrister. Then the judge was gone.

Of Neary, Justice Johnson said, "Dr Neary was very unconvincing in his explanations."

Allison had won. I left the courtroom and walked across the round hall. I rang Nicola to tell her it was over.

"And how is Allison?" she asked. I looked over towards Allison and Fergus.

"She is smiling, Nicola. She is smiling at last."

After Allison's case a lot of information started tumbling out like water from an upturned pitcher.

First there was the front-page story about the missing files in the *Irish Examiner* by Carl O'Brien. The other papers did follow-up stories.

I rang Bernadette in the records office of the Lourdes hospital. She was very nice and very helpful to me. She was very upset that she couldn't find the missing files. "They found one the other day and you should have seen the dancing around the place. I worked in records before and every file had links if it left the office so it could be traced. I am really upset about this," she said. "Do you think you will get an inquiry?" she asked.

"Don't know. The plan from now on is to get the women with no records to come out and tell their own stories. I am not going to be fronting it from now on."

"Yes, because these women are well able to tell their stories."

"I know. Especially now that Allison has won her case."

"Were you delighted with that?"

"Of course. It will all come out in the end and blame will be placed where it is due."

"That's only right. It's really heartbreaking for us too."

"I know, but you've been a great support to us."

I told her about a woman who had rung me the day before. "She rang the hospital twenty times and never got my number. In the end she got it from a journalist in *Ireland on Sunday*."

"That's awful," Bernadette said, with shock in her voice.

Then there were the revelations in *Ireland on Sunday*: the naming of the three obstetricians who supposedly supported Neary with medical reports in 1998. Frank Connolly wrote that the "three wise men" were Professor Walter Prendiville, Dr John Murphy and Dr Bernard Stuart. They were attached to two of the three major maternity hospitals in Dublin, the Coombe Women's Hospital and the National Maternity Hospital, Holles Street. Earlier in the year a Neary supporter had named these three men as the eminent doctors who had supported Neary. We distrusted information from that source. Did these eminent men really provide Neary with references, so to speak? It was these references that had made it necessary for the NEHB to seek an independent opinion abroad from Dr Michael Maresh.

When Jim Reilly next rang I asked him, "I wonder where *Ireland on Sunday* got the names of the three consultants? I didn't know their names."

"I don't know."

"Did they get the names right?"

"Well, those boys are very miffed this week."

"It must be true then."

"I suppose."

"I can't say I feel sorry for them then, but Neary probably told them lies. Or gave them very little information."

"Yes."

"Did you read the judgment?"

"Yes."

"The judge more or less said he was a liar."

"He did indeed."

Shortly after this a patient sent me a cutting from an article in the *Irish Medical Times* of 20 November 1992 – around the same time as Allison was in Drogheda hospital under Neary's care. The Chief Medical Officer, Dr Niall Tierney, was quoted as saying that the practice of foreign experts testifying in Irish courts in medical negligence cases could be challenged here. Objections could be raised to their evidence on the basis that they were from outside the jurisdiction. Their knowledge and sensitivities on local conditions would be imperfect. They may not be on the Medical Register in Ireland and on that basis alone their status as experts could be challenged.

This was six years before the NEHB was forced go abroad to obtain an independent review of Neary's practice in the interest of patient safety.

Katherine Cahill, a producer, rang on the Thursday morning after Allison's judgment asking if she would appear on *The Late Late Show* that Friday for ten minutes.

I said that she wouldn't; she had made up her mind and wouldn't change it, but I would ask. "Ten minutes is an insult anyway."

"It's just a teaser and this is *The Late Late Show*," Katherine said.

"I don't care. What happened in Drogheda is a national scandal – it's been all over the local radio in Meath. *Prime Time* made a great programme about it. This is off the record, but the women think he was doing it deliberately. And not only that, his mate, Shine, was accused of assaulting young boys in the same hospital for about thirty years."

"Say that again?" she said.

"You heard me. The women think he was doing it on purpose, removing the wombs of young women because he wanted to, and the national broadcaster is not interested. Public service broadcasting and all the rest."

"Are you serious? No one has been on to you?"

"No one."

"Leave it with me and I will talk to them here."

She phoned back that afternoon. She had twenty-five minutes to talk about it tomorrow night.

"Allison won't do it tomorrow night or any night. That's what she says, but other women might next week. This week is too soon. The women will want to talk to their husbands about it."

"Next week is the toy show but the week after. Can we meet and talk about this?"

"Okay; this time next week would suit," I said.

"I'll ring next week and we can arrange a date."

"That's fine."

In the meantime we were arranging the next meeting of the wider group for early December and new women still kept phoning. The numbers were approaching 100 by now. They included caesarean hysterectomies from women who lived in Drogheda at last.

After Allison's case, I had commented on local radio that only three women from Drogheda town were in our group. I didn't know why, but it must be significant. Drogheda people were not very supportive. Deputy Michael Bell didn't come to our meeting; the *Drogheda Independent* was not very helpful but they had apologised recently and that apology made all the difference to the women and was accepted.

After that, one of the Drogheda women agreed to talk to the *Drogheda Independent* anonymously. She was brilliant and brave for doing it. She threw up after giving the interview.

Katherine from *The Late Late Show* rang early in the week. We met at my house. She was an ordinary woman just like the women in our group. I thought they would like her. She could come to our meeting but I would have to mention it to the women first. The purpose of the meeting was to discuss the missing files and the statute of limitations.

By this time I felt that the next step for the women was for them to speak out more themselves. Otherwise they would never get the inquiry they so badly wanted. Also it was the next stage in recovery. Justice and influence were necessary to recovery and they needed to feel that from fighting their cause.

I said this at the meeting. There were a lot of new faces there, some old ones still. A long list of people willing to speak to the media was drawn up.

A further search was demanded of the NEHB to find the missing files. The number was growing now to between twenty and twenty-five missing files. Someone said that having no files made them feel like a missing person – a bereavement without a body.

Kathryn Quilty came, looking very vulnerable and frail, but she had her mother with her. Her solicitors came too, minding her.

Allison's much-loved dad died on the Sunday before the meeting, and on the Friday of *The Late Late Toy Show* she heard that Neary was to appeal – right at the last minute. At 5.30, notice of intent to appeal was served.

"Neary is going to appeal," she said.

After the meeting I rang Jim Reilly about a new search for the missing files. He told me there were developments in that regard. They could be going to the High Court to get permission to search Neary's house. There were rumours flying around that some people were getting panicky after recent media coverage and were spilling the beans.

The Late Late Show was amazing. I decided to wear black – Penney's best. I thought RTÉ was like a bunker with pale green plastic walls along its corridors.

Maria and Noeleen were on the panel. They both brought their husbands. Noeleen's sons came too. Special room was set aside for us. About twelve or fifteen of the women turned up. Jim Reilly came representing the health board.

Katherine said I would probably be asked questions and to remember "that passion and anger" I'd had at the meeting.

"I can't always be like that but I will try."

We enjoyed the show. Beautiful ballet danced by Monica and Roman from the Perm Ballet Company. Monica Loughman turned out to be a Dublin girl. I thought it gorgeous to see ballet so close up. Monica blessed herself about ten times in the wings before she danced. So elegant, so lovely, so beautiful in flowing sheer white.

Pat Kenny's introduction of the Neary story was frightening in its truth. "Imagine this. You are going into hospital to have a baby, full of terror at the birth, full of joy after the birth. Then this all turns to horror when you are told your womb was gone because you were bleeding to death. You believe this. You are grateful your life was saved as you were told. Then years later you discover it was all unnecessary. This is what happened in Drogheda."

Noeleen and Maria were magnificent as they told their stories. Noeleen read out the notes from her pathology report denying she had placenta acretia. She spoke so softly. Maria had been told she died. She had also been warned, from the beginning of her pregnancy, that it was likely to be risky at the end. Though she was perfectly fine, this worried her terribly. She didn't sleep well. After her operation her husband had told her what had happened. Neary had bawled him out, saying he could have killed his wife by telling her. She had died and he brought her back, Neary had told him.

Andrew spoke about how Noeleen would have loved more children. Caitlin, speaking from the audience, was gripping as she recalled how it was her baby who told her that her womb was gone – there was no cringing of the womb as she breastfed, she said. Majella, also in the audience, described how she was not told about her hysterectomy for ten weeks; how she told Jack; how they cried; how they thought it was their fault too.

Jim Reilly – Gentleman Jim – said that there was no box to tick for caesarean hysterectomy in the Institute of

Obstetricians and Gynaecologists' regular survey of procedures conducted in various hospitals, including the Lourdes. The procedure was so rare.

I saw a woman in front of me put her hands to her face and keep them there. There was total silence during the show. No cameramen moved; all was still.

Afterwards we went to have a few drinks. The men told me their stories. One moderate and gentle man told me how there was a hint of the butcher about Neary as he told him of his wife's operation all dressed in green, with a striped apron on him.

"Just for a split second it flashed through my mind. I didn't sleep for days. Neary told me not to tell her."

Katherine told us that all the anger came through on the show.

On the way home I heard a message from Cathriona. She thought it was brilliant; she was very pleased. Next morning Allison rang. She thought it was great too, and her mother was really pleased as well. Then Nicola rang. I had been worried that she would be broken-hearted past bearing. She had waited until the morning to watch it. She was okay and told me that what I said was fine.

A woman who hadn't even told her mother rang. She had watched it that morning with her husband and had been crying ever since. She had been crying for weeks, she said. This was probably a good thing, she said.

"I'm sure it is."

"My husband is beginning to think he was doing it deliberately. That was the feeling he got."

She cried on the phone, one of many crying today.

Jim Reilly told me that when he heard about Neary first, after the midwives confided their worries in October 1998, he had rung Professor Bonnar.

"How many caesarean hysterectomies have you done in your career?" Jim asked.

"One," came the reply.

"We have two in the last fortnight."

"Then you have a problem," came the answer in the sharpest Scottish accent.

He had a problem all right.

The truth was all over the place at last. And Fidelma Geraghty got in touch after the *Late Late*. She phoned me the day after the show.

"I couldn't believe what I was watching," she said. "The women were telling my story. I had heard of Neary and what he did but I felt it wasn't true of my case, that it didn't apply to me."

Then later, straight after she came to her first meeting, Fidelma rang again.

"I want to help in any way I can," she said. "I will do what is necessary. I have discussed it with my husband and have decided."

This was a godsend. Cathriona and I had been feeling the pressure. There were many women helping all the time, but Cathriona and I were the backroom women on an hourly and daily basis. Here was a great woman ready and willing to help at a moment's notice. After this, Fidelma and Cathriona would be central in going public for once and for all.

Dr Shine wrote to the Director General of RTÉ complaining about *The Late Late Show*. He said it was cheap TV; that vulnerable women were exploited; a good doctor was being destroyed. When I heard this I reminded Katherine Cahill of the other Drogheda scandal. "That's him," I said. "That's Neary's mate, the one who is accused of abusing boys."

Just before Christmas I got a phone call from a journalist saying he had heard there was a decision by the Medical Council's Fitness to Practise committee in the Neary case. Had I heard?

I hadn't and neither had the women. But maybe things were looking up.

On 19 February 2003, Niamh rang. Her solicitor had received an out-of-court settlement offer and wanted to know if anyone else had.

"It's the first I've heard of this sort of thing. Maybe it's because it's near court," I said.

"Yeah, I think so," Niamh said.

"How do you feel about accepting the offer?" I asked her.

"I don't know," she said, "but it would be all over. I could forget about it all."

"I know, and you are the only one who can make this decision. You're the expert on your own life, Niamh."

"Not really. I don't think I would like to accept it."

"They are probably afraid of you on the stand. You're a lovely young woman, the statute of limitations doesn't apply to you and you were one of the last to have a hysterectomy. They probably want to avoid the publicity."

During the next day or so I rang the other solicitors who were working on Neary cases. All said that the sum on offer was an insult, and none of their clients had received an offer.

I told Niamh's solicitor that the offer to her was the first, as far as I could make out.

"What sparked this off?" I asked.

"It just came out of the blue."

"It wasn't because you were ready for trial?"

"No, nothing like that. It just arrived in the post."

Next morning I rang Niamh again. I told her what the other solicitors thought.

"You haven't had a psychological assessment yet, have you, Niamh? All the women are affected. They are starting to have psychological reports prepared at this stage. You're bound to be affected too. Didn't we speak about it a few times before, that you shake sometimes, that you go white when you talk about it? I hope I'm not upsetting you, Niamh, but I feel I have to give you all the facts so you can make the decision that is best for you in the end. The offer does not include trauma. You need all the facts. I saw it in you, just like in all the other women."

"I've been finding it very hard recently," Niamh's voice went low. I knew she was suffering greatly.

"You wouldn't be human if it didn't affect you, Niamh."

"I haven't phoned Allison."

"Why not do that? She is dying to talk to you. By the way, I didn't tell anyone who'd got this offer. Only the amount."

"Can I tell Allison?" Niamh asked.

"Of course. Allison can be trusted to keep her mouth shut."

Niamh laughed. "I'll get back to you again."

She was beginning to come around.

The following week I got an email from a patient I was supporting about a totally separate issue. She had been in contact with the Medical Council with her own complaint. She wanted to know the result of her inquiry. She was told it was up to the doctor to decide whether or not the patient was told the result of an inquiry.

Then I remembered that the Council had written to a few women some time after Christmas. They were informed that there were no findings of professional misconduct against Neary in their cases. This information came out very slowly and referred at that time to one of our women, Noreen. Naturally, she was very upset, as was her husband, but we provided her with support. We knew how she was hurt. Rumour reached us of other women who also received this result but they were not in our group at the time.

I wondered if that is why they were told? It was in Neary's interest to tell if there was no bad finding. Did this mean that there were findings against him in the rest of the cases? Significantly, was there a finding against him in Niamh's case? Was that why Niamh was offered a settlement out of the blue?

Next morning I rang Cathriona and told her of my suspicions. She and Jenny rang the Medical Council. They were told that the Neary inquiry was over. They got the very strong impression that if they had not been written to there was a finding against Neary but that the official result would not be available until after the next meeting of the full Council, probably in May. In the meantime, the Fitness to Practise committee would be reporting to the full Council.

22

The Supreme Court Finds for Allison

On 1 May the hearing of Neary's appeal against the High Court judgment in Allison's favour was heard in the Supreme Court. The appeal was purely on the grounds that too much time had passed for Allison to sue. There was no appeal on negligence.

Allison's barrister was certainly put through his paces. He argued that Allison did not know sufficient facts to seek legal advice. She knew only that her womb had been removed. This could not be considered damage because, as far as she was aware at the time, it was done for the purpose of saving her life – or so she thought. Otherwise, any patient who had a hard time in hospital would in future have to go to a solicitor as they leave hospital. Neary's barrister worked very hard, citing several cases in support of his view that she was barred from taking the case. The exceptions relating to time referred to secret illnesses like asbestosis and hidden cancers, he argued. Not medical negligence.

I was shaken after this hearing, not at all certain of success. So were many of the women. Allison was very upset, though her solicitor said she was happy with how things had gone in court. Other lawyers said there was anxiety round the Four Courts about the outcome. There was an expectation that Allison would win, but it was by no means certain.

The maddest week of all started with Allison's phone call on 1 July. I was in Lisbon. She was very nervous but the decision was due on Thursday at 10.30 – the day I was flying home. My holiday was over after her call. People had to be contacted. I texted everyone. By now we had a network established. I could text Cathriona, Nicola, Maura, Fidelma, Niamh, Rosemary, Róisín and Teresa, and in about half an hour most of the 100 or more women in our group would have the latest news. Cathriona would be on the phone too.

On our last day in Lisbon we toured the city, its shopping streets and its sights. I had to keep my mind off things. We had wine in the Rua Augusta in the afternoon. I wondered how Allison was. My reservations about the outcome of the appeal became fear now. Allison and Fergus must have been in bits.

Next morning, as Allison waited with Fergus and their legal team in the Round Hall of the Four Courts for the appeal decision, Cathriona and her mother arrived with Justin and Seamus, Cathriona's two boys. Justin was about twelve, but grown-up for his age. He quietly approached Allison, tugged gently at her sleeve and said "Good luck", concern in his voice and on his face. Justin was about the same age as Allison's son.

271

Later Allison would tell me how Justin's gesture tugged at her heart as she walked in to hear the court's decision. She knew her boy was worried too. She thought of him.

Unfortunately, my plane was late that morning – about twenty minutes. I turned on my mobile as soon as it landed, at 10.40 a.m. There was a message for me but I couldn't hear it. It was from Cathriona. I thought the doors would never open – ten minutes that stretched from here to eternity. In the aisle, I finally heard it at 10.50. She had won.

Wilfie threw his arms around me. I had to get a taxi quickly. There was another call from Cathriona and one from a journalist. I would meet them at the court. There we met Maura and Pat, as well as Cathriona's mother and her two kids Justin and Seamus.

She couldn't text me, she said, her hands were shaking too much. I understood; mine were too. RTÉ called. We all went out to Donnybrook. I was very nervous doing the interview for the *News at One*. Very emotional.

Allison rang in the afternoon saying she loved the interview. She had cried when I mentioned her name. How relieved she was it was all over. She would do no interviews; her days before the cameras were over. How could she do interviews, she joked – wasn't Mary Wilson too gorgeous anyway?

Despite the joy, there was real sorrow and relief that day. It was a low-key day, really. Not an anticlimax; more a feeling that it was the beginning of the end. I got my hair done in the afternoon. Allison rang the next day too. She was heading to Cork with Fergus and her son. She was still smiling.

"We took a huge risk but we had no choice. And didn't I beat him clean?" she asked.

"You wiped the floor with him," I said.

Cathriona and I were busy over the weekend too, talking about the next meeting. There were loads more phone calls and more women were helping, gaining courage from Allison. The fear of saying something wrong was gone, the fear it would not work out all right.

Conor Ganly, a medical journalist, told me he had a copy of Harry Whelehan's report into the Medical Council's office procedures. "There are only four copies in existence. The Council doesn't like it. It backs up all you said about their procedures – no system, letters unacknowledged, unanswered for a considerable length of time, insensitivity, etc. The Council is saying it is very legalistic," Conor said.

"That's good, coming from them," I said.

The following week, Allison was awarded her costs. The smile was still on her face. "I'll never forget what James Nugent, my barrister, said to me. He said I made history and whatever else they took from me, they can't take that. I beat him, didn't I?"

"That's for sure, Allison."

"Anyway, it's all over," she said.

I told her about our next meeting. "I wouldn't miss it," she said. "And there were still some people saying I will never have any luck with that money after what I did on him."

"Take no notice of people like that. There are always people who don't think straight."

Then I told her what Jim Reilly said, "The boss said 'Yes!'" when he heard the result of the appeal.

"They'd have been in trouble if I'd lost too."

"They surely would."

And Deirdre Gillane rang on Bastille Day. The Minister would meet the women any time; just let her know and she would arrange it.

At our next meeting in the Boyne Valley Hotel, Allison spoke to the women about her case. "You should have no fear of going to court," she told them. "I had medical questions answered by Mary Wingfield and John Bonnar there. But the judge in his ruling told it all to me. The judge was the one. This was sorted for me in the judge's house, the place where you just tell the truth. The rest took care of itself. When you are there, just remember that you are in the judge's house," she explained.

She described the healing power of the court, of telling your story, of seeing the truth written down in black and white afterwards. "Then you move on and give up the bitterness," she said. "I am a new woman."

She had told me earlier that she kept asking Fergus if he liked his new woman, the one who was smiling all the time, the one who told him to go and play golf if he liked. There was no need for him to stay in and mind her. She looked great at the meeting. The women thought the same. "She looks taller," they said as we sat around afterwards.

Allison left after a question-and-answer session. The rest of us were sitting in the lounge, finishing a cup of coffee, when my mobile rang. It was Allison.

"You'll never guess who I've just seen," she said.

"Who?"

"Neary, stopped beside me at the traffic lights. I said to Fergus coming up to the lights to mind the fellow coming up behind us. 'He's very pushy and driving funny.' We had to give way to him. I couldn't believe it. It was him, looking like a down-and-out, in his '94 LH car, a coat-hanger for an aerial. He looked straight at me, as close as you and me were tonight."

"My God, he is still round the town then. Did he recognise you?"

"I don't know. I just thought I'd tell you."

"Thanks," I said. "But how did you feel?"

"I just thought, isn't that incredible? Fergus and I were amazed." Allison's voice was light and amused. No sign of pain. That was the healing power of bearing witness and giving testimony.

That was how the day ended.

But everyone was still annoyed with the Medical Council and the Minister at the meeting. It had been almost three years to the day since Micheál Martin had come to a similar big meeting. I told the women of his invitation to see him in September. This time there had to be results, not just sweet talk and soft eyes. He had hurt Nicola, she told me the next day, because she had believed him at the very first meeting. She didn't know if she could meet him again; he had done nothing to monitor how the Medical Council did their business. He was weak, she said; she couldn't trust him, he had hurt her too much.

We took policy decisions too. The women wanted a public inquiry and a tribunal of compensation. There was a new feeling of strength. Something had to be done about the hospital, about it as a supposed centre of excellence, about inquiries behind closed doors. I asked for volunteers to talk to the media and I got them.

I was sorry that our doctor, Tony O'Sullivan, was not there to see this. He deserved to be. He had left day-to-day work in Patient Focus to devote more time to the Diabetes Federation at the beginning of June. A Neary supporter had complained about him to the Medical Council under Fitness to Practise for his role in supporting the women. Seemingly, a part of the Council's Ethical Guidelines required doctors to support each other. Clearly, Tony came down on the side of hurt patients! The Medical Council process would take a few months. I believed it was a vexatious complaint. The women and I were all very sad about Tony's departure, but completely understood his reasons. In the end, the Medical Council decided Tony had no prima facie case to answer.

Ita's Story

Ita's story was astonishing. She had an incomplete miscarriage and Dr Neary arranged for her to undergo what is commonly called a "D and C", a minor surgical procedure usually done on a day surgery basis. Certainly that is what Ita expected when she consented to the procedure.

However, when she awoke she discovered she had undergone a total abdominal hysterectomy, with the removal of both her ovaries and fallopian tubes. She had not given consent for this surgery; it had not even been discussed. She expected to go home to her husband and children that evening. Instead she found she had undergone major surgery.

Dr Neary told Ita he could not stop the bleeding. Later, she was told she did not have cancer. None of this was discussed with her. Neary noted on her files that he thought she had advanced cancer of the womb when he operated.

This was not the only such case and is one of the worst abuses he perpetrated on women. What she had was a miscarriage, and Neary removed her womb and ovaries. In that strange unit, no questions were raised after this extraordinary operation.

23

The Medical Council Decides

On the last Friday in July, Wilfie and I were in the car on the way to the ballet in the National Concert Hall when Susan McKay from the *Sunday Tribune* phoned.

"Can we talk?"

"I'm on my way to the ballet, Susan. What is it?" I knew it must be important but hoped it wasn't.

"I've just heard that the Medical Council is going to release the outcome of the inquiry into Neary next week. I heard he was found guilty."

"What! From who?"

"A reliable source. It's definitely true. Well, the Fitness to Practise committee have found him guilty but it has to go before the full Council. I'm told they never change the decision of Fitness to Practise," she said.

"Oh, they do sometimes." I knew of a case where this had happened.

"But not this time, I'm sure. How could they?" Susan's calm, steady voice reassured me.

"Oh yeah, I know, that's great."

"Can we talk in the morning?" she asked.

"Yes, of course, I'll be home. Any time. Thanks for telling me."

We had just arrived at the ballet. We had a joyous evening and a lovely meal after in the coffee house there. I didn't sleep.

The next day I heard from Susan. Neary had been found guilty of ten counts of professional misconduct. It was to be released to the media on Tuesday.

Everything ends, I thought, *even this*.

I rang Cathriona (who was in the airport), Nicola and James. We couldn't get Noreen but she rang that night. I texted Niamh, Allison, Emily, Noeleen. I was texting and talking all day. But it couldn't come out. We had to keep it to ourselves for a few days.

Later I would learn from Cathriona that this was the worst of all days for her. She could no longer hide the awful truth from herself, even momentarily. If they struck him off in her case, it must be very bad indeed. She didn't enjoy her holiday. She carried the grief to a beautiful Portuguese villa with her.

On the Monday, I asked Allison if she would like to go public, as when the news broke she would surely be asked.

"I don't want to go on the radio. I have done my bit but I want you to say for me that I am a new woman after my case; that I bear no ill will towards Michael Neary; that I am grateful to the Health Board for the respectful and confidential way they treated me, in particular Jim Reilly, a real gentleman at all times; and finally, I believe there is now sufficient reason for the Minister to set up a public inquiry and a tribunal of compensation for the other women."

She went on, "I could see the pain on the women's faces at the meeting last Wednesday. I could recognise it because it was me up to very recently. All the women deserve the resolution I had, but some haven't the strength for court. Dr Neary destroyed himself, it wasn't me that did it. He allowed himself to self-destruct by what he did and continued to do."

The news broke on Tuesday, 29 July, just as Susan said. I caught it on the 4.30 p.m. headlines on FM104. Just minutes before, I had spoken to Nicola. The Council had, just moments before, told her that nothing would happen until the following day, so I was relaxing, or trying to.

I was immediately on the phone to Nicola again. "It's happened. I heard it on the news. He's been struck off."

"What? Are you sure?"

"I'm certain."

"And they just told me it would be tomorrow. Isn't it a terror?"

"How do you feel?"

"I don't know. I never thought it would happen."

"Well, it did. He's stopped now," I said.

"Will you get on the blower and begin telling everyone?"

We all phoned, texted and talked for the rest of the afternoon, trying to get to as many of the women as possible. Nicola, like all the women, was pleased but very sad.

After the Medical Council's decision, every TV and radio station and newspaper in the country wanted to talk to a "Neary woman". Some of the journalists who called at that time were too pushy. They had no understanding of what it cost these women to talk. One got the feeling that they personally just wanted to be as high up on their news programmes as possible.

The Medical Council had also expressed its sorrow to all the women concerned for what had happened to them in Drogheda. This was a very special and fulsome apology on a very special day indeed.

On 20 August it finally became clear that there was no possibility of Neary appealing. Jenny rang the Medical Council and the offices of the High Court. No appeal had been filed in the High Court or served on the Medical Council, she discovered. It had been flagged that way, but no one believed that he wouldn't appeal.

I rang Nora Owen for advice and help. She had been solid before. The best thing was to get a date to meet with the Minister, she said. She would encourage other TDs to write to him asking for a public inquiry.

On Wednesday 19 August I received an email from Jim Reilly. I could not believe its contents: an apology from the Medical Missionaries of Mary to the women. An apology which had not been sought. It contained no ifs or buts either.

The women had to be told before it was made public the next day. I got on the phone. Most of the women were stunned – ten seconds' silence and then the gut feeling. Some were angry, saying it was too little too late; others felt it was better late than never. All were grief-stricken, it opened everything up again, but it was better that it happen than not – especially for the women in Drogheda town. Only a seriously deranged person could disbelieve them now. Also, the nuns called for an inquiry. But there was no mention of the word "public". I hoped that the nuns would personally take media calls. They didn't.

Paul Maguire was coming to my house the next morning to do a training video with RTÉ. He had just started to work there, having previously been the LMFM presenter who first drew me in to the Neary story five years before. After consulting some of the women, I told him of the apology. They wanted him to know. He was always fair. When I showed him the press release, he asked me to do an interview about it.

"Okay, right, but you must guarantee that it will not be shown until after the apology is made public."

"I give you my word."

"Right." We did it.

By then I was really tired and pleased to be going to a friend's for lunch. On the way I heard the apology on the 12.45 p.m. news on Today FM. It still shocked me to hear it. I was on the motorway, so I missed my exit. I drove around for the next hour but at last I found my friend's house with its beautiful garden. I enjoyed a brilliant lunch from a wonderful cook.

The nun's apology was the lead on RTÉ's *6.01 News* and again at 9.00. Paul's lead story was great for the women.

One of the women rang next day. As a result of the news report, she had told her little boy.

"How did the doctor treat the wounds?" he had asked her as the item rolled.

"No, love, that's not it. He took out wombs, not treated wounds," she said. She had to tell him. She told him she was one of the women, just like Allison.

"I will never forget his face," she explained. "He went from confusion to some understanding very quickly."

"Is that why I have no brothers and sisters?" he had asked her.

"Yes."

"Now he is sad," she told me. "He is quiet. He is thinking."

"We must do something for the kids."

"When is this ever going to end? They have a lot to be sorry for in Drogheda," she said, quietly as usual, referring to the nuns' apology.

The Health Board agreed to fund counselling for the kids if they wanted it.

On Wednesday, 27 August, the *Irish Medical Times* web page reported on a decision by the Medical Council to publish their report on the Neary inquiry and to give the women involved a copy of it two days beforehand. In addition, they were to refer it to the Gardaí. This was unprecedented and greatly appreciated by the women. Despite the long delays, the women felt it came right in the end. I felt this very much too.

RTÉ's *Morning Ireland* rang looking for a reaction. All I could say was that I didn't have any words. I was stunned. I would have to ring the women.

Nicola wrote the headlines for the news the next morning. "It was what we always wanted but never dared wish for," she said when I rang her to tell her the report would be referred to the Gardaí. This was the first time ever that I heard a tone of justice creeping into her voice. She wrote the statement that I read out to the reporter, Will Goodbody. *Morning Ireland* led with her reaction on Thursday morning.

These were her words: "The women and their families are very glad that the Medical Council report into Michael Neary is to be published and forwarded to the guards. They are stunned that at last someone has taken notice as to what really happened in Drogheda. It is what they have wanted but dared not wish for. They say that something like Drogheda must never happen again. That is what is most important now. They agree with the Council that a full and broad-ranging public inquiry must be held into all the serious outstanding issues pertaining to the hospital. This is necessary so that lessons can be learned and applied to all areas of medicine. Only in this way can confidence and trust be restored."

I went into the *Morning Ireland* studio, where I was interviewed alongside Professor Gerard Bury, President of the Medical Council. Off-air, he worried about the women receiving the reports.

"They will be all right; they have each other," I said.

"They have you too," he said. He looked down at the ground. "I am not trying to flatter you," he continued, "but you deserve a lot of the credit for this."

I was taken aback. I knew then that the Council had suffered too, had had their own difficulties with this awful story. He explained what would happen. The following Tuesday the Council would go to the High Court to have Neary's name removed from the medical register and then immediately the women would be sent out their copies. We hadn't even asked for this. Furthermore, Professor Bury supported a broad-based inquiry into what happened. He felt ashamed to be a member of the same profession as Neary, he told me. All negative feelings I'd had melted away and were replaced by respect.

On the airwaves, Professor Bury called on the Minister for Health to take over from here. It was up to others to take it further. There was a need for a broad based inquiry.

Minister Mary Coughlan was sitting in the studio as I left. I couldn't miss this opportunity – a government minister, a social worker by profession, a woman too. I voiced the need for a public inquiry. She hummed and hawed; public inquiries are very expensive, she told me. I went into overdrive explaining to her the need to examine the hospital to get answers; I felt no empathy coming back to me. But even that did not burst my bubble.

On 2 September 2003, Michael Neary was finally removed from the Medical Register by the High Court. The next few days were total madness. The phone never stopped ringing – new women, other patients too and, of course, journalists. The women were finally able to come out in public. The ten women whose complaints had been upheld also received written apologies from the Medical Council.

For me there was a sense of completion, a relief, an exhaustion. From that point on, it was what happened in the hospital that mattered. The role of other professionals needed to be looked at; why did they not stop the abuse?

Meanwhile, all that the Minister of Health was talking about on the media was a smoking ban – a smoke screen! The day after Neary was finally struck off, Micheál Martin was on the radio talking about smoking. Not a whisper about Neary.

But the doctors of the Medical Council were still talking and being quoted in *The Irish Times*. They wanted monitoring of doctors, they said. Professor Tom O'Dowd was quoted as saying: "The report shows the medical profession 'had its own bad eggs'. If a doctor wants to do damage like Shipman or Neary, the system is still of such a nature, because it operates on trust, that it is possible for a doctor to actually start off doing an awful lot of damage. It's that nature of a job and the art and trick of the thing is to actually pick them up early. And where there is data available it's got to be scrutinised . . . and there's also got to be peer review and audit."

The doctors supported us.

The Medical Council published the report of the inquiry into Neary on 4 September, at a press conference, a day after the ten women had it delivered to them by courier. It was very traumatic. Cathriona showed a copy of it to RTÉ news; again, they led with it at 9.00 am. She went on *Morning Ireland* too.

Katie and I went to the press conference. I didn't know if we would get in; I wasn't invited but I wanted a copy of the report. A journalist told me the time and place, but when we got there we weren't sure if we had things right. We parked nearby and skulked around to see if we could sneak in without anyone noticing. If we saw cameras, then we'd know it was on. Sure enough, at about 2.50 p.m., I spotted Robin Boyd, the RTÉ cameraman, as he walked down the road to put money in the meter.

"Can we go in with you?" I asked.

"Course you can. Aileen O'Meara is here with me."

"They won't throw me out if you're there," I said.

"It's Aileen they'd be afraid of," he said.

"It's you too and your camera," I said.

We got in the door of Lynn House, having identified ourselves as from RTÉ.

"Remember when we started here three years ago?" I asked Aileen.

The place was full of journalists. Everyone was there.

Professor Bury spoke eloquently, saying that Neary had damaged women, families and babies. It must never happen again. A review of the Medical Practitioners Act 1978 was well overdue.

I asked if Neary had been psychiatrically assessed. "No, we can't do that under the Act."

The need for competence assurance, a process whereby doctors can verify that they keep up to date with developments in medical practice, was put forward. It was down to the Minister to establish it on a statutory basis.

I asked about the involvement of Drogheda women in any future Council under a new act. "We need more lay people," was Professor Bury's reply.

A journalist asked if they supported a public inquiry. The gist of the reply was that they supported an efficient, effective, broad-based inquiry.

Professor Bury told the press conference, "The report is to be referred to the guards very shortly."

At this stage the women were still in fighting form, but depressed too, because everything they suspected had been proved true, written down in black and white by the doctors' report into one of their own.

I visited Nicola in her house. Her report made for shameful reading: a tissue of lies by Neary; altered notes too. As we looked through the report, a Neary supporter was on local radio. The denial still went on, just as we were unable to believe we had succeeded.

The day before my visit to Nicola, the last remaining teenager not to contact us had phoned. She was just nineteen when Neary removed her womb at the birth of her first baby. "He removed my womb," she said quietly, "but there was no stress or anything. He just said to my husband, 'I'm losing your wife.' Neary never told me for a week or so. He just came in, tipped me on the toes and said, 'No more babies for you', and walked away. My files are missing too," she added. "I've tried to get them from the hospital but they can't find them. They have my file number but no file."

24

The Trouble with Public Testimony

The first of several meetings with the Minister took place on 23 September, a bright, sunny Tuesday afternoon. From our point of view, its purpose was to request a full statutory public inquiry into the obstetric and gynaecology unit of Our Lady of Lourdes Hospital back to 1974. Nothing less would do.

Coincidentally, in the previous Saturday's paper, the long-fought-for legal notice – that Michael Neary had been removed from the medical register – was published. On an inside back page. "Imagine how things could have been if we didn't campaign," said Cathriona. "That is all there would have been, if even that. He might not even have been struck off at all." And she might have been right. The mood among the women was that sticking together would get us everywhere. It would make sure it never happened again.

"A public inquiry gets all the stories in the open. People are asked awkward questions. No one reads the final report anyway. It is the public telling that matters," Cathriona believed.

"That's all we want. Pray for it. I've gone off religion recently since I read Neary was a very religious man. But maybe I can go back now," Nicola said. "Is it too much to wish for? Everything has gone our way so much recently."

"No, it should happen," I said.

Allison was really optimistic. She rang the day before the meeting with the Minister. She was certain he would immediately announce a public inquiry.

I was doubtful. "He has never said a word in public about this whole affair yet."

"He is going to make a statement tomorrow and that will be it," she replied.

Lots of women wanted to come on the day to meet him. We trooped to Bewley's: Cathriona, Sandra, Róisín, Noeleen, Andrew, Fidelma, Orla, Teresa, Maura, Una, Sally and me. We ordered chips and sausages or buns and tea.

The first hurdle was to make sure everyone met the Minister. I rang Deirdre Gillane. "There isn't enough room; we can only cater for seven," Deirdre said.

As we got to Hawkins House, lights were flashing, cameras rolling in the bright sunlight. A few of the women got out of the way of the cameras.

In the end, we negotiated for eight women and one man to go in. Having to select those to meet the Minister was terrible. This was new and very painful. It seriously affected our mood. They kept us waiting in the conference room for forty-five minutes. A civil servant came in once to apologise. I phoned Deirdre again. "Is the meeting going to be today, Deirdre?" They were sorry; they would be there soon.

Finally, they all trooped in. The Minister shook hands with everyone and introduced his team, six or seven of them, including at least two legal advisors, one from the Attorney General's office and one from the Department of Health. I introduced the women and Andrew, who would represent his mother Noeleen.

Cathriona opened the meeting proper. She came out straight: "The women need a public tribunal."

The Minister spoke about the difficult current climate surrounding tribunals. The proposals of the Minister for Justice Michael McDowell for statutory but less expensive inquiries were in the making. Tribunals were expensive; there was a public mood against them; they filled the pockets of lawyers and went on far too long, he explained. The message certainly was that we've had far too many tribunals in this country for our own good.

Cathriona joined in, firmly speaking of the need for professionals to be questioned in public. So did Andrew and Fidelma.

"The McDowell system of commissions of inquiry held in private can give people the chance to tell their stories," Micheál Martin said. This was under consideration by the government.

"But the women need answers," Cathriona said. "We want to know why this went on for so long and why no one did anything about it."

"It is even more important than the story telling that the professionals give public testimony," Andrew said.

Fidelma added her views too. "This could be happening in other hospitals now. We need to publicise it to make sure it isn't."

"How wide is this going to be?" the Minister asked. "We could open a can of worms here. It would never end. That's what happened with the organ retention inquiry; it went far too wide."

We stated the range of damage in the whole unit: young women who had their wombs and sometimes ovaries removed after having their first or second baby; young women in their twenties and thirties who had their ovaries removed unnecessarily for minor gynaecological problems; then there were the older women profoundly damaged by unnecessary gynaecological procedures; and not forgetting the two grief-stricken women whose babies died in very worrying circumstances.

"We want a judicial inquiry covering all these issues. We have said it over and over again. Everyone knows it," Cathriona said.

"A fundamental aspect is the public element. We have always made that clear as crystal," Fidelma said.

Cathriona then brought up the missing files and placed the need for a compensation tribunal on the table.

"I am in favour of an inquiry," the Minister said, "but I need to put it to government. I wanted to talk to you before I did that, to see what you wanted. I will look into that and we can meet this day three weeks."

The meeting lasted a long time. All our cards were on the table. Fidelma prepared the statement for the press. By now most had gone home. We were all pleased.

Two or three days after the meeting, all hell broke loose on the radio in Drogheda. People rang in saying things like, "It was all for money", "Neary was wonderful," he delivered their babies, etc.

We had moved on from Neary; he was history. The focus was now on the hospital. The strong possibility of an inquiry was now in the public domain. Some people, it seemed, were very worried.

The women in our group were worried by the local reaction. A form of paranoia grew up amongst them. They went on local radio to defend each other. They cried sorrowful tears. Fear was everywhere. I rang the show's presenter to tell him. He said there was a view out there in Drogheda that resented the inquiry. He wanted to show it for what it was. It was time for the women to look after each other again.

A short notice case pushed forward by Neary's solicitors brought Rosemary Cunningham's case to the High Court suddenly. It was a statute of limitations case, and the question again was, did she or did she not know? And if she did know, for how long did she know? Should she have come to court earlier? These were the questions. The judge was Aindreas Ó Caoimh. I thought he was a decent man as the hearing went on, though he terrified me to start.

Rosemary and Eugene, her husband, got a week's notice. Her barrister was very blunt as he explained to them standing outside the courtroom what the consequences of losing would be – €50,000 down, it seemed. There was the usual messing before the case got going – would there be a judge free and a court free, who would it be, when, would we have to come back the next day all over again? After lunch we heard it was going ahead that day.

There was legal argument about detail of the pleadings. When that was resolved Rosemary gave her evidence as to what had happened to her, how Neary abused her verbally, how she could not forget it for a long time, how he removed one of her ovaries. As the case went on, I grew in strength. So did Rosemary and Eugene. The time in the witness box was excruciating for her. She found it very difficult to tell her story. She was pale, and she broke down once or twice. But she was great.

The TV coverage was very explicit that night. The papers the next day reported it too. Rosemary was appalled by it. She was afraid the court would think she had given an interview because some of the information reported came from her affidavit, not from what she had said in court. We reassured her the next morning that this was all right.

Neary's barrister questioned her very closely, the same question over and over: how much did she know when she wrote the letter to the Medical Council on 19 December 1998 about the removal of her ovary? She reiterated that she did not know that the removal of her ovary was unnecessary until Dr Porter's report in May 2000. She told the court that her main complaint to the Council was about Dr Neary's verbal, not physical, treatment of her. She acknowledged that she had not suffered as the other women had physically. Nevertheless, she wanted to tell of his barbarism. She wanted to stand up and be heard. She never would have pushed this all the way to a court hearing. Neary's side selected her case from the large number outstanding at the time as a sort of test of the statute of limitations.

Rosemary rang to ask us to emphasise to the Minister at our next meeting that the women must be protected from court, but must also get a public inquiry. At mass on Sunday, she was shunned by some people; one woman pointed her out on the street. Three came up to offer their best wishes.

"It is a very small place where I live. Only about 150 people go to mass on a Sunday there. I wasn't going to go, but Eugene said, 'You have nothing to be ashamed of,' so we went. They might think I'm washing my dirty linen in public, or that I am looking for money. I am not going to get much out of this – my solicitor explained this to me – but it's important this comes out."

"Are you sure you still want the public inquiry?" I asked. I wanted to be sure she hadn't changed her mind after her recent experience.

"Oh, it has to be in public," she said still. "Tell the Minister that the women must not all be taken to court; it is all very terrible. But the truth must be exposed."

Some of the women rang to say how delighted they were that Neary's verbal abuse of them was coming out in Rosemary's court case. I passed these messages on to her.

True to his word, we met the Minister again on Thursday, 23 October. By that time we had formed a committee to represent all the different strands of injured women within the group. Cathriona, Fidelma, Maura, Orla and I met the Minister in his office this time. It was a much smaller meeting in a lovely spacious room with comfortable sofas in the outer office. The Minister had two officials with him.

He had been to government and they were agreed on the need for an inquiry.

We restated the need for the staff of the hospital to give evidence in public. We told him what Rosemary said after her hearing. This was not vindictiveness, it was merely asking questions, just like Rosemary was asked last week in the High Court.

"I know it's not vindictiveness, but it would be seen as such by the staff of the hospital," he said.

"Probably," Cathriona said, "but they would be wrong. We also need to get all the damaged women in. It needs to be broad-based, like the Medical Council said."

"This could open floodgates," said the Minister.

Towards the end of the meeting he told us, "We have approached someone eminent to head the tribunal."

We were surprised it had taken so long for the Minister to tell us this.

"Is it a household name?"

"I can't say yet. They are involved in other things and have not yet given their response to the approach."

We still thought we would get a full public inquiry in the end.

In October 2003, Dr Shine stood trial in Dundalk Circuit Court for allegedly indecently assaulting six teenage boys between 1974 and 1982. Shine denied the assaults, which were alleged to have taken place in either Our Lady of Lourdes Hospital or at his consulting rooms in Fair Street, Drogheda.

A number of his former medical colleagues gave evidence that Dr Shine was very thorough in his clinical examination of patients. Some nursing colleagues gave evidence of working with Shine and none had ever received a complaint about him from a patient (*Irish Times* Report, 23 October 2003). Dr Shine was acquitted of all charges. However, a

Medical Council Fitness to Practise inquiry recommenced into similar allegations concerning him.

Tuesday, 28 October 2003 began nervously. We all hung around outside Court 14, because other business was being dealt with first. It was 11.30 by the time we got in. The view was that Neary's team might have a victory that day. There were lots of barristers hanging round. There was a lot of interest in the judgment.

Justice Ó Caoimh read it out, so it took some time for us to be sure. He decided in Rosemary's favour. She did not have sufficient knowledge until she got the report from Dr Richard Porter. It was from then that the time started to run. She could sue.

The next day the papers carried pictures of a smiling Rosemary. She had not slept for two weeks but she was smiling.

25

A Judge is Appointed

We had the third meeting with the Minister in late November. This time we were given tea and scones in the canteen in Hawkins House. The meeting had been postponed at the last minute a week before. The women had been on the bus to Dublin at the time. We were all dressed up and nowhere to go. We were given no explanation except that "the Minister couldn't make it". So Fidelma drafted press releases, we went to the media and complained. It got a small outing on the one o'clock news. Maybe that's why we got the tea.

The Minister apologised for the postponement. "Due to a court appearance," he said.

"What worries us," we told him, "is that you have never made a statement in public about the Neary affair other than to say you were moved and were looking at options."

"I have said I was appalled." He raised his voice. He leaned over towards me. I was sitting next to him around the table in his inner office.

"That's what the women feel. We can't deny that," I replied. I didn't want things to get too hot and bothered.

"We intend to appoint Judge Maureen Harding Clark to chair the inquiry," he told us. "She is in the International Court of Justice – the Yugoslav tribunal."

"That sounds very good, but we just don't know," Maura said. "We need time to look into everything."

"I haven't heard of her," I said.

Now he looked at me disapprovingly.

"We will have to look into it," someone else said.

"You are not going to criticise her in public?" asked the Minister.

"Of course not," I said. "We are just wondering who she is and what her credentials are – you would be the same. We will look her up."

"It will be a non-statutory inquiry with a small public dimension – the women will be able to tell their stories in public," he said.

"I am very disappointed," Fidelma told him.

"We got your terms of reference," the Minister said. We had forwarded terms of reference that covered all the injuries at the unit since 1974, gynaecological and obstetric. He looked worried. Was this the "can of worms" he had mentioned earlier that he didn't want opened? "We have not produced any yet," he said.

We emphasised the importance of including every damaged woman and of investigating the missing records. Fidelma's records were missing, as were several more women's.

"Our legal advice is that those without records can take cases too," the Minister said.

"Yes and no, Minister. Our advice is that it is hard enough to take a medical negligence case with records – never mind with none."

Cathriona reiterated, "We don't want to be locked out of this inquiry like we were at the Medical Council. And at least they came up with the proper answer."

"We must take this back to the wider group," the women said.

Afterwards in Bewley's we compared notes and expressed how disappointed we were. We spent the afternoon writing to the wider group. We invited them to a meeting to discuss recent developments.

I told Wilfie about the judge. He emailed me with her details in no time. She certainly sounded very impressive. I began to focus on the positive, on all we had achieved since the last meeting with the women after Allison's case. There was the Medical Council decision, ratified by the High Court; the nuns' apology; Rosemary's case; referral to the Gardaí. Now we had the promise of an inquiry too and a judge appointed. All we needed to do was to agree terms of reference, develop the public aspect and set a timetable.

That indeed was what was agreed at our next meeting with the full group. There was a huge turnout. People kept coming. The meeting agreed our motion to accept the judge appointed by the Minister, to pursue further the public aspect and to involve in the inquiry all women damaged in Our Lady of Lourdes Hospital's maternity and gynaecology units, regardless of doctor or procedure.

We met the Minister and his officials again just before Christmas. The Christmas mood was everywhere. We discussed the terms of reference, restating our need for wide terms that included all damaged women. We all agreed that the format be parked for the time being. That stumbling block regarding private versus public hearings could be returned to when other matters were agreed.

Seemingly the judge had already started work. I understood that the NEHB had written to the Minister too, recommending a public inquiry as were we. The Minister also told us he was giving us funding of € 10,000. And we hadn't even asked for it! Christmas had come early; best wishes and good will prevailed.

A few days later the disks of the full Medical Council inquiry into Michael Neary were with Nicola, just two days before Christmas. But Nicola was great. In the last week too I heard that a Medical Council inquiry into Dr Lynch, the other obstetrician at the Lourdes Hospital, was to open on 8 or 9 January. There was only one complainant to a full hearing, and we had been looking after her all along. That was a very satisfying end to the year.

While we were waiting for Dr Lynch's case at the Medical Council, it was covered by the medical press and picked up by local radio and other media, including RTÉ and *The Irish Times*. This was May's complaint, which the Medical Council mislaid and which led to the Whelehan review of their office procedures earlier. But it did not go very well for us. There was no finding of professional misconduct.

In the first week of the New Year, though, a tiredness returned to us all, a New Year syndrome. But this year was worse because my husband was very sick, laid low by the flu and not recovering. I had to take a back seat.

Fidelma and Cathriona were filling the void I left very well. Cathriona received a letter from Neary's solicitors saying that the Medical Council decision in her case had no legal binding on her High Court civil case and so they would not proceed to an assessment of damages. No surprise really. But we also heard news of a court lodgement of € 140,000 in one woman's case.

We met the Minister for the fifth time at the end of January. The media knew about it and turned up at Buswell's Hotel as we got together to meet the Minister. Wilfie was still very sick and not getting better either. (It took several months for Wilfie to recover completely.) I was very worried about him, so Fidelma gave the interviews before and after the meeting.

"He is always in a good humour when we meet him here," Maura said, referring to our meetings with the Minister in Leinster House.

"Hope the mood is good today," we all said.

We were not kept waiting for long this time. "They are beginning to talk about us now, not having thought about it since before Christmas," Fidelma said as we reached the office. Everyone agreed. Out of sight, out of mind was what we felt.

The meeting was brief by previous standards. Micheál Martin was like a different Minister this time; he's a man of many personalities and sides. This one took control of the agenda.

He told us they had prepared draft terms of reference, but they couldn't show them to us. ("They won't, they mean," we said to each other later. We even wondered if the papers before the Minister on the table were terms of reference at all.) "They were with the judge. They must go to the Attorney General first. Judge Harding Clark has appointed two lawyers and is looking for premises. She says the inquiry terms of reference will be based on the Medical Council inquiry. That is what is possible legally." The Minister's tone was soft and polite as he told us that only caesarean hysterectomies would be inquired into. It had to be ring-fenced. There would be no inquiry into the removal of ovaries from young women and older women; nothing about the baby deaths either. So no cans of worms would be opened; ring-fencing was secure.

We were horrified and told him so. Orla told the story of her baby's death. He shuffled. The others were silent.

"And there are the older women too," Maura pointed out. We went over the same ground: all injuries must be included; evidence had to be in public.

"We will talk about these things with the judge," the Minister said.

Fidelma again asked for the terms of reference. He refused again. "I can't give them to you," he said wistfully. "You will have another meeting with the officials in a week or so," he said, ending the meeting. "They will be in touch."

Afterwards we expressed our alarm. "We have been downgraded to officials and nothing is agreed with us," said Cathriona.

"You said it," Maura agreed.

We gave a holding statement to the media after the meeting. We did not say that we really felt we had been let down. We were very depressed.

"We are never going again without lawyers," said Cathriona. "They have taken advantage of the fact that we were willing to negotiate by ourselves. They've had their lawyers, haven't they?" We all agreed.

It was Orla's intervention that turned the meeting a bit, after she told them about her baby. Maybe they would look at things, they started to say towards the end. They would discuss it with the judge. We consoled ourselves with this.

In late February, the medical press rang. "I hear from the Department that it is going to be a private inquiry," the journalist said.

I filled him in, saying that the women would not co-operate with such an inquiry. There had to be a public element and a broad-based approach to include all the different strands within our group. I told him we would trust the judge to decide what could and could not be in public. *Irish Medical News* ran with the story that Patient Focus would not co-operate with a private inquiry. This was followed up by *The Sunday Times*, where an unnamed official was quoted as saying we had been threatening to withdraw all along. That was not true. Our clear view all along had been that we would walk away from a fruitless inquiry, but we were eager to be innovative in our approach. We always understood the Minister's need to save money and we had wished to work with him to develop a new kind of inquiry that would suit all of us. We had always said a large part needed to be in public, but clearly everyone was entitled to due process.

Meanwhile, day after day Fidelma was ringing the Department of Health civil servant Denis O'Sullivan to put pressure on about the terms of reference. I don't know how she stood it. Eventually they turned up, faxed to her on Friday 5 March, at four o'clock. She rang me straight away and we opened them together, so to speak. She read them out to me.

The first clause was disappointing, too narrow. It referred to obstetric hysterectomies only. No abusive gynaecology was included, and no baby case was included. I rang Maura and Orla. They were not surprised. We would keep going. We were very upset for Orla.

The second clause appealed more. It involved a detailed examination of the processes in the hospital – who spoke to whom, if anyone did. But there was nothing about the missing files, no examination of what happened to so many women's files. And it did not seem to go all the way back to 1974, when Neary joined the hospital.

"These papers are the nearest thing to cabinet papers," the official had stressed to us. "They are highly confidential."

We were not going to betray them. Mine came in a brown envelope, stuck all over with sellotape. We would think about it the following week – consult our legal advisors, the inquiry's legal advisors and the women – before we made a decision. As if that decision was ours!

26

A Limited Inquiry

We met with the judge's advisors in Bow Street on 23 March 2004. We all gathered in the round hall of the Four Courts first. As usual, all of us came. This time we also brought our legal advisors – Colm, Hugh and Senior Counsel Dr Michael Forde. We walked in convoy to Bow Street and the grey building at the back of the Distillery complex that was to house the Lourdes Hospital Inquiry.

Fidelma, who had worked so hard to get this meeting and the terms of reference was the first to notice the sign on the door. "Look at that," she said. Everyone stared. It read:

COMMISSION ON ASSISTED HUMAN REPRODUCTION

"Not a good omen," Fidelma laughed.

"Jesus, that's amazingly insensitive," someone else said.

"Maybe they will be offering IVF inside, or surrogacy advice," said Cathriona.

Rob, the office manager, eventually came to the door. Our legal advisors joked and talked on the way down. Michael Forde's trousers were amazing; hadn't seen an iron in a while, I'd say. His shoes were worn too. Yet he stood taller than the rest of us.

"It's great we won't have to do any talking this time," I whispered. "We can rest."

Inside it was a typical civil service building: green plain carpet; magnolia walls. Rob said he would show us around the building where the Lourdes Inquiry would be held. He showed us the interview room – clinical enough, I thought, but adequate. But I felt worried for the women who would be coming in here to tell their stories of how they were deprived of their fertility, of their femininity in some cases, and of their relations with beloved partners.

Michael Forde asked for a minute to talk to his clients, to be briefed by them. The women told Michael what they needed: the terms of reference were too narrow; the public element was missing; there was nothing about the other damaged women or the missing files, etc. They decided to go the whole hog and ask for a full public statutory inquiry again. Everyone was agreed on this. And the lawyers would do the talking.

We were ushered into the big boardroom – a large dark wooden table in the middle, about twenty comfortable leather chairs around it, water for everyone. This was feeling better.

After a short while the civil servants and inquiry lawyers joined us. Paul Barron, a senior civil servant, sat at the top of the table with his civil service colleagues, Deirdre Gillane next to him. On Paul Barron's right sat the inquiry's legal advisors, then the women with our legal advisors.

Fidelma said she wanted to say something on behalf of the women and as a victim of Michael Neary before we got into discussion.

"The women were very hurt by the plaque on the wall. They think it very inappropriate and insensitive."

The new arrivals looked confused.

"The Commission on Human Reproduction plaque on the outside wall," she explained.

Paul Barron reacted. "It's not my fault. We don't own the building."

"I just want to make that point," Fidelma said.

Someone else explained, "I think they were here, but are on the verge of moving out now."

"It could have been covered up," Fidelma emphasised. "We can continue with the business now. I just think that needed to be said."

Paul Barron chaired as the most senior civil servant there. Everyone introduced themselves. The atmosphere was pleasant and cordial all the time. Then the judge's legal advisor, Kevin Feeney, spoke. "This is a private non-statutory inquiry," he said. He filled us in on the background.

Everyone had the terms of reference in front of them. Michael apologised for being late; he needed a cup of tea after a case. He put forward the need for broader terms of reference. Other procedures had to be included. He had our list – babies who died, ovary removal, gynaecology damage. Compellability of witnesses was important too.

Colm said the inquiry title should not mention Michael Neary by name. Hugh said that the women wanted to hear what other staff at the hospital had to say.

The meeting went on for two hours. It was cold in the room. Kevin Feeney, the inquiry's legal advisor, explained that a hybrid inquiry was not possible. Paul Barron said, "The government and the Minister have decided the inquiry is not to be statutory. The matter was ended." He closed the meeting with a profuse apology both for the plaque and his reaction to it. His apology was accepted.

Afterwards we went for a drink, despondent. We got nothing we wanted. Anger at Micheál Martin was very high.

"His meetings were just a PR exercise. He never listened and he was very rude too," Maura said. They could conduct the inquiry without us. They probably would.

Michael Forde calmed the situation. He felt that they were open to extending the terms of reference. We could get other things, possibly, such as compellability.

"How important is it that Neary gives evidence?" he asked.

"Very important," was the unanimous reply.

Next day I phoned Maura at about 10.00 a.m. "I'm flaming mad," she said. "We might even have to march. If that's what it takes, that's what it takes."

Fidelma was also very upset. "If I ever thought I was anyone, I didn't after yesterday. I felt like a lump of meat. A piece of dirt."

I had never seen the women like that before.

Later that week a journalist from *Irish Medical News* rang. "Neary is not going to give evidence unless made to. What do you think of that?" he asked.

"Nothing. Neary is sorted," I said. "The only thing that would bother me is the possibility that he can reapply for admission to the Medical Register." One of our women had received a letter from the Council saying they would hold her complaint on file in case he made such an application.

In the midst of all this, "New Guidelines for the Medical Profession" was published that week, containing a lot of what the women wanted. Professor Bury, the President of the Council, was all over the newspapers, pushing reform. We had achieved a lot. We should celebrate. There was an editorial in *The Irish Times*, too, the likes of which I thought I would never see. Didn't we do well!

On the no-smoking day, 29 March, Micheál Martin, our Minister, had a victory breakfast in Bewley's. He was riding high, smiling on worldwide TV. He was being hailed as a great Minister for Health, almost like Noel Browne, or Donagh O'Malley in Education.

He gave an interview to the medical press. He was to bring in a statutory patients' complaints system. There was to be no statutory inquiry into Drogheda, though.

I was asked for our reaction. Had we not always called for a full public statutory inquiry? "In public, that is our very strong position," I said. "But in private we were hoping the Minister and his Department would be innovative. We were aware of the public mood towards tribunals and of the public purse. That is why we kept faith with the process. We were ever hopeful. But we are angry with him now. He has dishonoured the process, as has the Department of Health with the terms of reference they produced."

We were told that the terms of reference were in the public domain. And we thought they were top secret. This was reported the day before we were to meet the Minister again on 5 April.

The wider group was horrified by the inquiry that was on offer. Some of the men offered to protest, to walk to the Dáil. But we had to keep going. There was a piece too in that morning's paper about how unhappy we were, followed by pre-recorded interviews with the Minister and me on the lunchtime news. I had agreed to be interviewed after talking to Fidelma.

On radio I said we could not accept the terms of reference or the lack of compellability. Neither Neary nor the women would be giving evidence at this tribunal, it now seemed. Instead, it would be a civil servants' and lawyers' inquiry.

Allison had offered to come to this meeting. She looked very beautiful and relaxed.

The Minister was in a talkative mood. We found it hard to stop him. But we did. We had spoken to most of the women. They had made up their minds not to co-operate.

"What happened since the last meeting?"

"Nothing. We are still of the same view as before."

"We never agreed to anything," Fidelma reiterated.

"All the women have to be included and there has to be compellability. The women feel disrespected by what is on offer," Cathriona said.

The tone was quite rude and defensive, on both sides. But the Minister did not seem to want to go.

"I told Denis O'Sullivan very clearly we would have no choice but to walk away," Fidelma said.

"The terms of reference are what were discussed at the meetings."

"No, they are not," she said. "How can you say that?"

He said again, "They are," getting redder and angrier all the time.

"Well, we must have been at a different meeting," I said.

The Minister made suggestions as to how the impasse could be got over. Orla spoke about her baby again, how the focus was too narrow. We needed the right of anyone who wanted to give evidence to be copper-fastened. Guarantees from the Minister, however well meaning, were not enough. It was not in his gift.

Also, we needed compellability. Allison expressed our worry to the meeting. "Only two of the ten people in theatre the night I had my baby were in the court to give evidence in my case: Neary and me. No midwife could be found. They would not give evidence voluntarily."

The Minister agreed to go to cabinet with our needs. He would get back to us in a couple of weeks. Afterwards Fidelma spoke to the media, saying we had a positive meeting. It went out on the 6.01 and 9.00 p.m. news. The Department issued a statement saying matters had been clarified.

Allison was amazed at how we had given out to the Minister. "Such a lovely man," she said.

On 26 April a letter arrived from Judge Harding Clark, detailing her appointment on 6 April as judge to the Lourdes Hospital Inquiry. She described her willingness to talk to anyone but emphasised the starting point of the inquiry, which further narrowed the timetable to the 1990s, and the focus of the inquiry as peripartum hysterectomies. This meant that a small number of the women who would have been excluded by the strict interpretation of the caesarean hysterectomy procedure would now be included. Peripartum hysterectomy covered any woman who had her womb removed within six weeks of the birth. This eventually covered a very small number of the women who we had previously classified as a gynaecology case.

The judge's tone was gentle and conciliatory. She would talk to any woman who wanted to speak to her. She asked for my help in encouraging people to assist the inquiry to find the truth by asking them to start preparing statements. There was no mention of compellability. She also said she would be advertising soon.

I was not surprised. Fidelma had spent the previous week getting in touch with people like Deirdre Gillane, trying to set up another meeting with the Minister. There were no return phone calls. It was now a *fait accompli*. The women felt totally betrayed.

The judge's letter was dated 6 April, the day after we had met the Minister. What about his promise to go to cabinet with our difficulties, to get back to us?

Three days later, on 30 April, Linda rang to say that Neary had been found guilty of professional misconduct in her case, and in two more cases. After the original inquiry, a number of other cases had been considered by the Council. Very little attention was given to this and some of the women concerned were surprised but pleased when they were invited to give evidence. Patient Focus supported the women who needed it, as before. The matter was over and done with much more quickly than the original inquiry. Linda, however, was very upset. I was worried that if Linda was upset, then everyone else was in real trouble. I emailed everyone to tell them.

On 4 May we sent out a press release.

Patient Focus is very sorry to announce that the women and families it represents cannot take part in the Lourdes Hospital Inquiry. The Minister Micheál Martin and the Department of Health have, in its view, behaved in bad faith towards us. The inquiry announced falls so far short of what is needed, that the women have no option but to decline to participate. This is because of the narrow terms of reference and total lack of compellability of witnesses and documents. The women have decided that the pain involved for them in giving evidence is too great for what is on offer.

Allison emailed, again expressing the view of all the group. "I am very disappointed. I can't believe how that so-called Minister wasted all our time. It is lovely the way the government protects the professional person and not the ordinary person. If there is any more I can do, let me know."

We felt we had no option but to withdraw from the inquiry. We were mirroring the Minister's behaviour. Micheál Martin was "disappointed and surprised". He would of course meet us again. As a response to our press release, the Minister said he had offered a meeting and we had refused. In fact, he offered the one timeslot we told his secretary we could not make. We needed a meeting with the women. It was no longer enough to talk to them over the airwaves.

The numbers were growing too; there were now 170 women or even more.

The inquiry barristers also wanted to meet us again. We met them in the Airport Hotel. Jim Reilly set it up and came too. We talked for three hours or so, everyone having their say. The barristers answered our questions fully about who would be covered by the inquiry; only caesarean hysterectomies. That was it. At the end of the meeting, they understood what would be missing from the inquiry if we didn't participate. We told them we believed the Department of Health and the Minister were to blame.

27

Kathryn and Rosemary

In mid-May too, solicitor Gillian O'Connor rang to say they had reached a very good settlement for Kathryn Quilty. Kathryn had been only twenty when her womb was removed, in January 1996, by Neary. That month he had performed six caesarean hysterectomies. Cathriona was very upset to discover that she and Kathryn were in the hospital at the same time and did not know of each other. Would I come to the High Court to support Kathryn the next day? Of course I would.

"I'm meeting her and her Mum in the round hall at 10.30 a.m. We'll meet you there," Gillian said. We talked for a long while. By this time, Kathryn was in a flat in Drogheda with friends. She was fine.

Next morning I arrived early in the Four Courts. Kathryn and her mum turned up at about 10.00. We looked at each other from opposite sides of the Round Hall until her solicitor turned up at about 10.20. I wasn't sure it was

Kathryn; she looked different. She looked absolutely wonderful in her cream jacket and black trousers. She had filled out and was now slim rather than gaunt. Her hair was healthy-looking too. And her mum was with her. My hair had turned grey, which is probably why she did not recognise me.

On the radio later, after her case was settled, I heard Kathryn say she would buy a little house for herself and her son and learn to drive so she could take him out for spins, because he really enjoyed that. She wanted to talk, though, to do something for others. I was amazed she was so strong telling her story, dignified and powerful. She got a great reaction in Drogheda, where she lived. When she and her mum went out, people hooted their horns at them and put their thumbs up. We felt this was a significant change and probably now meant that people who had quietly supported the women all along or who merely had an open mind on the matter up to this now felt free to express their views.

"It was great," Kathryn said later.

On 17 May there was a huge attendance in the Boyne Valley Hotel by the wider group. Another date, 20 May, was set to meet the Minister too. Kathryn came with her mum. She had a gift for me. I was dying to open it but couldn't there and then. There was a top table this time. The committee, one by one, briefed the meeting about the lack of developments and how unhappy we were. Having briefed the meeting, we broke for tea. We asked each table to elect a representative to tell the committee of the results of its deliberations. Should we co-operate or not? In the event of non-cooperation, what would be the next step for us? We needed suggestions.

One after the other the tables said that under no circumstances should we co-operate. In fact, they said it was time for a protest march unless Micheál Martin came up with something more. The meeting decided we would arrange a press conference on the Tuesday following the next meeting with Micheál Martin if we were not happy with what transpired. People were very eager to demonstrate – even outside the hospital. The committee thought this would be a terrible idea; the press conference in Buswell's Hotel would be better. We decided on this. They would all come to Buswell's on the following Tuesday if necessary.

When I got home I opened Kathryn's gift. It was two beautiful glass dolphins, blue and white. Kathryn wore a silver dolphin round her neck that night. Today her gifts sit on my windowsill at the turn in the stairs. Kathryn's media intervention that week was a turning point for the wider group. She provided another example for quiet women that telling your story could be done with great dignity.

Before the meeting with Micheál Martin, Deputy Liz McManus phoned. "Be careful of totally boycotting an inquiry," she said. "They will just go ahead anyway and you will be well and truly shut out." We desperately did not want that. A way would have to be found.

Jim from the NEHB was also worried. He spoke for an hour with officials the night before. He told me too that the midwives who had revealed Neary's misconduct had dates to talk to the judge. "We are getting co-operation from others too," he said. This information was a help.

Before the meeting, tea, coffee and biscuits were provided for us. We had great fun with Allison and her good form set the tone. There was no need to be difficult today; we were just to listen and then implement our press conference option. Those were our instructions from the wider group: to put serious pressure on the government.

We brought our solicitor this time. At the meeting Colm again pointed to the main issues – compellability and the inclusion of other procedures. We mentioned too that we were worried that the Medical Defence Union was now talking about refusing indemnity to the women and negotiations with the Department had broken down.

Eventually the Minister said a government decision had been taken to constitute a commission of inquiry under the McDowell proposals, which would allow for compellability of witnesses and cross-examination too under a statutory framework, if there was non-cooperation by hospital staff. Would that solve our compellability difficulties? Stories of women who were damaged in other ways would inform the inquiry report, he said, including the women whose babies died. They could be interviewed as part of the process of investigation. The report, we were reassured, would be frank and full and published. These promises were put in writing shortly after the meeting. They kept us in the process.

The appeal into the High Court decision in Rosemary Cunningham's case was heard on 15 June 2004 in the Supreme Court's Hugh Kennedy Room. Hugh Kennedy was a former Chief Justice, we discovered from portraits on the wall outside it. Portraits of other Chief Justices were there too. I saw Justice Keane's portrait on the gallery wall.

Several of our group turned up – Cathriona and her mother Anna, Maura and Pat, Fidelma, Noreen, brave after her husband's recent sudden death, and me. Rosemary looked well. "I don't have to give evidence this time; just watching now," she said.

Rosemary joked with her barrister, Michael Forde, about the hard time he had given her before she gave evidence. He knew he had. "Aren't you glad I did? You turned out to be a great witness," he joked back.

Today, Justice Hardiman presided with Justices Fennelly and McGuinness. No one ever knows when we might have to walk into one of these rooms, waiting for justice to be laid out in front of us, wishing it was a jewel that glistened and could be seen and touched and weighed and admired. But it is not like that. It is dull and tedious.

Neary's barrister talked in a low monotone, arguing why Rosemary knew, saying that she must have known if she had written the letter to the Medical Council. She was therefore, he argued, out of time.

Then Michael stood up and said he had never heard of a particular point just made before. "How can you say that? It is in the submissions, is it not?" asked Justice Hardiman. I thought his tone was judicially assertive.

And so they went on, sparring back and forth, looking for a moment in time, a eureka moment, on which to pin Rosemary's awakening of knowledge. This date and that were mentioned: the time of the initial publicity, referred to as rumour by Rosemary; the time the nurses told her to write to the Medical Council; the date she received the medico-legal report. Did her GP's opinion that nothing was wrong medically last until the second legal report? Points were scored on both sides, over and back, over and back. It was like receiving heavy blows to the jaw during a heavily fought boxing match for us. We felt things were going against Rosemary. She felt ill and had to leave court for a while. The case lasted the day. Judgment was reserved.

At this time, the Minister for Justice, Michael McDowell, was busy putting the Civil Liability and Courts Bill 2004 through the Dáil. He proposed to reduce the time limit to file a medical negligence claim from three years to one. Very strong arguments were made in the Dáil about it from all sides. Patient Focus made strong representations about the difficulties this would create for damaged patients. Minister McDowell eventually relented a little and reduced the period from three to two years.

In the first week in July, the inquiry advertised. They had kept in touch with our group and our confidence was growing day by day. The solicitor to the inquiry had phoned to say that we could drop in at any time. Furthermore, in the guidelines I read that women could bring a friend, family member or solicitor with them while being interviewed. That was very good news. It didn't happen in other inquiries that I knew of.

Richard Dowling had an item about the opening of the inquiry on the RTÉ news. We saw the look of Judge Harding Clark, dressed in a smart pink suit. "Looks nice" was the general verdict. I had told them of the gentle tone of the letter she sent me and of its contents. They were prepared to give it a chance to succeed because of this.

"A woman I would talk to," Nicola said. "I listened to see if I liked her voice."

"And did you?"

"I did; I will go to the inquiry."

"That's great," I said.

Women were phoning to say they had made appointments to tell their stories to this judge, in whom they were placing enormous faith. Everyone felt really excited about it.

On 2 July I rang Deputy Caoimhghín Ó Caoláin and asked him to raise the status of the Garda inquiry into the missing records in the Dáil. "Nothing has happened in relation to the Garda inquiry. There were rumours a little while ago that there would be news. It came through a journalist but nothing happened. Can you find out for us?"

He asked for details and said that it was the last day for raising questions before the Dáil broke up for the summer. He promised to ask the Minister for Justice and send the reply to me.

On Wednesday, 8 July, Maura gave her evidence to the inquiry. I was anxious to hear how it went as she was the first woman interviewee of which we were aware.

"It is the first time I have felt good about any of this," she told me. "It was a very good experience. I would have been very annoyed with myself if I hadn't done it."

"It is great to hear that," I said.

"It makes me feel more confident when recommending to the other women to go."

On that day Jim Reilly asked to meet me as a matter of urgency. We met that afternoon. The Gardaí wanted to meet me, him and some others the following week to begin preliminary investigations into the missing records. Perhaps that was a result of the parliamentary question, I thought. We did meet with some very senior gardaí the following week. After that meeting, I knew that those men would do their best. They asked for my help in getting a small number of women involved to progress the case.

As life arranges, the mother of a dear friend of mine was being buried on the same day as Rosemary's judgment was due. I got texts from both Fidelma and Cathriona while I was in the cemetery in Shanganagh: "Rosemary lost the case"; "Neary's side won"; "All three judges went against her".

I spoke to Rosemary about thirty minutes later. "I am devastated but holding up. Everyone is here with me and that really helps," she said, referring to the women who had turned up to support her. Fidelma said that she knew from the look on Justice Hardiman's face that we had lost. Cathriona said they mumbled, "Appeal granted".

The Supreme Court decided that Rosemary's knowledge ran from the time she had written the letter to the Medical Council, about Neary's appalling rudeness to her, in December 1998. Her letter referred only peripherally to the fact that he had removed her ovary.

As usual there were loads of interviews, this time with Fidelma and Rosemary. On the TV that night Rosemary looked beautiful in defeat and in pink – "A suit I bought for a wedding," she said when I mentioned it. They called for a tribunal of compensation for the women who were out of time, in terms of the statute of limitations, and without records. Minister Martin said he would examine the judgment and denied that he told the women at an earlier meeting that his legal advice was that the statute of limitations time would not run until the date Neary was struck off by the High Court. Rumour and a letter to the Medical Council could start the time to run.

Jim Reilly reassured me that the NEHB had a senior counsel at High Court hearings because the Medical Defence Union was defending the action. Otherwise, if the MDU won, he explained, the Board would be left with the liability if they had not defended it too. It could be assumed that they accepted liability by not contesting the case.

This explained why the health board senior counsel attended all the hearings and merely commented from time to time that he agreed with Mr Meenan's points. Mr Meenan was senior counsel for Neary and his insurer, the MDU.

Come September we had arranged a meeting with Enda Kenny, the new leader of Fine Gael. Cavan/Monaghan TD Seymour Crawford set this up. We wanted to brief Enda Kenny on Rosemary's case and seek Fine Gael's support. As usual the women came – Cathriona, Anna, Fidelma and, of course, Rosemary and Eugene.

Seymour was there at 4.00 p.m. as arranged but Enda Kenny did not turn up until about 4.30. He was accompanied by Olivia Mitchell. We made the point that a redress board was needed for the Drogheda saga to reach a just conclusion. People like Rosemary would otherwise be excluded from obtaining justice, and not just because of lapse of time. Her complaint was about unnecessary gynaecological surgery and she was not covered under the strict terms of the Lourdes Hospital Inquiry, although Judge Clark was speaking to women like her.

"Is there an Inquiry into the Lourdes?" asked Olivia.

"Yes, it's been up and running since April and is going very well," I said, flabbergasted that the opposition spokesperson on health did not know this after all our efforts. And she was one of the sympathetic politicians.

We emphasised that Liz McManus and the Labour Party were very supportive, as were people like Deputies Jim Glennon and Mary Wallace, and we wanted a commitment that the need for a redress board would be part of Fine Gael policy. We were also going to discuss this with the Labour Party and the Greens.

"We won't engage in auction politics," Enda Kenny said. "Every group has worthwhile objectives and we cannot say yes to everyone. What I will do, though, is raise the matter at Taoiseach's question time when the Dáil has settled down after the reshuffle. As leader of the opposition I will have two minutes and I will raise it then."

That was all we were going to get. We emphasised that we were going to make it an election issue in the forthcoming by-election in Meath following John Bruton's departure as European Ambassador to the US.

The following day on the train I heard from a journalist that Neary was one of the obstetricians the MDU was refusing to cover.

I was interviewed by the Inquiry on Wednesday, 22 September. Many of the women in our group had given evidence by then, as had Jim Reilly. The Inquiry had been very quick to respond to my phone call, much quicker that I expected; in fact, within a couple of hours I had my appointment. It happened to coincide with Aideen's debs that evening, but no matter; better get it done.

I was interviewed by Senior Counsel Kevin Feeney and Judge Maureen Harding Clark. It was a long interview but the tone was amiable and friendly – more of a chat. They asked about the origins of my involvement with the Drogheda story, if I had any connections with the town, and how Patient Focus emerged. I told them of my interviews on LMFM at the very beginning; the visit to the NEHB in Kells with Nicola and James; how we developed from six women through to sixty or so by the end of summer 1999; the fact that we got medical reports first, then legal advice. I described how Patient Focus was established as a legal entity, that we had an accountant, that we now had an office since this summer. I was now paid a salary but, at the start, everything except hotel rooms for our meetings and some money for phones and stamps was paid for by Tony O'Sullivan and me. I told them how we had been afraid to take funding in the beginning from the Health Board, but that we had grown to trust them, because they put services in place for the women.

I told them too of the needs of the two women whose babies had died to be heard at the inquiry. At a meeting of the wider group the night before in Drogheda, I had learned that Sandra had received a letter saying it was not intended to talk to her at present. She was very upset about this; as was Orla, who had not been written to but was told on the phone it was not within the terms of the inquiry. Kevin Feeney said that perhaps they could ask a paediatrician to talk to them and explain what happened to their babies. I wanted this as soon as it was suggested.

We broke for coffee as I was telling them of my shock at the medical reports coming back in September 2000 and of Dr Clements' comments to the women. Judge Harding Clark said this was the first they had heard of this.

Like the women, I felt listened to there. By now, more importantly, most women had told us they felt the process had been very healing for them, including the women whose complaints were gynaecological rather than obstetric, the young women whose ovaries were needlessly removed, plunging them into severe and very early menopause, as well as the older women.

The Gardaí were getting very interested. We had asked them to examine the missing records. We met them in Drogheda during August. Introductions were made and people were amazed that things were on the move. We had a second meeting in the Boyne Valley in October at Garda instigation. This time, several senior gardaí turned up. Many of them were in the vicinity because of the recent Rachel O'Reilly murder in North Dublin. The solicitors came too. Niamh came. I could see one of the gardaí's eyes follow her around the room as she came in with her mother, so shocking was her youth. We were totally convinced of the seriousness of the Garda approach after this meeting. We were told of the personal interest of the Commissioner in the matter. "If he is interested, we'd better be," a senior officer said.

The following week, the Gardaí raided the homes of Michael Neary and a local Drogheda woman. A journalist who lived nearby saw the whole affair. So it was on the front of the *Mirror* the next morning.

"Neary was very nervous," we were told. The Garda raids discovered copies of some of Fidelma's and Celia's records, but no originals in his house. Copies of other missing documents turned up there too. Nothing was found in the woman's house.

In the end no charges were brought in relation to this. Judge Harding Clark in her report found that the files were stolen, but no culprit could be clearly identified. The Gardaí explained that the failure to discover any original files in the houses, along with the lack of a proper signing-out process for records in the hospital, prevented the DPP recommending charges. The DPP decided that there was insufficient evidence as to who was responsible to allow charges.

28

Floodgates and Ring-fences

A number of the civil legal cases were settled during 2004, including Cathriona's, Nicola's and Linda's. Settlements were in the main between € 100,000 and € 150,000, with one exceptional case receiving € 200,000. After the Cunningham case, however, the situation became much more difficult for the women and their lawyers and the case for a redress scheme to be established by the government became compelling. There were a number of reasons for this legally:

- As a result of the Cunningham decision, all summonses issued after December 2001 were challenged on the grounds that they were out of time, as three years had elapsed since December 1998, when the Drogheda scandal became public. This defence was raised in almost all cases, even though many women were not aware of the problems with Neary until much later. While this defence could be overcome, it caused great stress for many of the women.

- A significant number of files were missing. By now we knew it amounted to thirty-nine at least. Obviously complaints about unnecessary operations cannot be proved without files.

- Expert witnesses were raising questions about atrocious record-keeping and even altered records. Proving records had been tampered with requires the level of proof of a criminal trial. Clearly this was very difficult for the women.

- Solicitors for the Medical Defence Union were no longer taking instructions in cases involving Michael Neary. Clearly the only option then was to sue the doctor personally.

- A judge of the Supreme Court, Justice Hardiman, raised the issue of fraudulent misrepresentation against Michael Neary in the Gough case. This would defeat the statute of limitation defence but on the other hand the insurers would not have any obligation to cover the doctor if fraud were involved. In relation to criminal assault, the same difficulties would arise, with insurers likely to refuse cover.

In addition, the number of cases that were being settled out of court, mainly women who'd had caesarean hysterectomies in the mid- to late 1990s, was drying up. Reaching a settlement out of court was a very humiliating experience too, with women describing the process as leaving them feeling dirty and further abused. One woman couldn't even remember how much she had received.

"How much compensation did I get?" she called to her husband when I spoke to her on the phone one evening.

"€90,000," he replied.

"I just wanted it all over," she explained to me. "I couldn't look at the cheque when it came. I told my husband to put it away for the children. That's what I did. I never handled it."

This issue needed to be tackled. The women wanted closure. They needed to move on with their lives. Trauma was making it difficult for people to talk about their experiences.

Not counting caesarean hysterectomy, we estimated the numbers amounted to twenty-five people in all – hardly floodgates. We knew that the women who did not have caesarean hysterectomies were particularly vulnerable to being excluded from any scheme. It was these women who elicited the phobias of cans of worms, floodgates and ring-fences. It was, we felt, the reason for their exclusion from the inquiry proper and the reason for the strong efforts to confine the inquiry to the findings of the Medical Council. We would mention their plight at every possible opportunity.

Such an opportunity – to speak publicly of the need for a redress board – came knocking on our door. A news report in *The Irish Times* in October related a "leak" of confidential documents from the Inquiry. Legal advice to the NEHB relating to the legitimacy of using a private detective in connection with the large number of missing files at the hospital was among the documents inadvertently released. *The Irish Times* saw this advice.

This leak caused huge distress to the women. If this had been a statutory inquiry, providing the press with such information would have been an offence. As it stood, the judge could do nothing; there was no comeback.

I spoke to the judge. She apologised and explained how the leak had happened. Documents that were used for an interview were all contained in one folder. When asked for the return of documents related to the interview, the legal advice was mistakenly sent as well. It was clearly a very serious breach of security. The story was also carried by *Irish Medical News*.

"The leak is a diversion," we said. We used it as an opportunity to talk about the need for redress. We were going to write to Mary Harney and request a meeting with her, as the new Minister for Health, to discuss the need for a Redress Board. I took the opportunity also to speak of trauma, missing files, statutes of limitation and the pulling of indemnity by the insurance company. At this time too, garda involvement had the effect of focusing minds. People at last knew the seriousness of this. This allowed me to mention the possibility of doctored records as well as stolen/missing records. National and local media picked up on this.

In the run-up to Christmas we prepared the ground for redress by inviting all the local public representatives to a meeting with the women in January in the Boyne Valley Hotel. By the start of the New Year, we were confident we had the support of Fine Gael, Labour, the Greens and Sinn Féin and several Fianna Fáil deputies. By now, there was still no support worth talking about from Ministers Noel Dempsey and Dermot Ahern, though the refusals were definitely getting more polite. Phone calls from pleasant-sounding people were now coming to our office, rather than a mere letter stating that they would be out of the country or a brusque brush-off from those answering phones to the women.

There was still nothing much from Dr Rory O'Hanlon. He was now Ceann Comhairle. He was precluded from coming to a public meeting but would meet people separately in his constituency, he said.

We were canvassing candidates in the forthcoming by-election in Meath too. Sirena Campbell was selected at convention by the Progressive Democrats as their candidate. We invited her. She was young, pleasant, bubbly and honest. She would come to our meeting. The Labour candidate Dominic Hannigan couldn't make it but Sean Ryan would be there and Dominic would send a representative. Ministers Dermot Ahern and Noel Dempsey didn't do that. Brendan Smith rang to apologise. We reminded him that he hadn't been able to come the last time either, because of a back injury. He was surprised we remembered. We invited Mairead McGuinness MEP, who phoned personally and was very nice but seemed not to know a lot about the situation. This worried me given her age and gender. She was, though, very willing to listen.

"I hear both points of view about Dr Neary. Some of my friends found him to be a very good doctor. But I know what he has done. How can there be this disagreement?" she asked.

"If he damaged every woman he would be out of the hospital in a week, don't you think? It would have been obvious wouldn't it?" I remarked.

She went silent for a moment and in a way that made me realise she was listening, and seriously too.

"That's true," she said.

"Did you have your babies in Drogheda?" I asked.

She said, "No."

I said, "I'm glad."

A very helpful woman from Deputy Jim Glennon's office phoned several times, trying to contact the Minister for Health's office for us. No sign of our letter from 8 November could be found, they told her. I knew they had got it because I had spoken to a senior official in the Department at a conference in December.

"Your letter is being considered but the Minister won't be contacting you in the near future," he had said. "Her personal style is different from the former Minister's."

I explained the upset of the women and I sensed irritation on his part. I pressed him about when we could expect to meet her.

"Not in January anyway," he said.

"That will really upset the women and their families," I said.

Mary Wallace, very hospitably, met the women in her home. She phoned the same senior official while they were with her. When was the Minister going to meet the women? His attitude to her was no better, they gathered from the tone of the conversation. She had asked for a briefing twice already and had not received one, she told him. "There isn't one," we believe he said. Mary Wallace told him that was an inappropriate way to talk to a member of the Oireachtas.

In the end we invited a small number of the media to our meeting. But we asked them to keep it completely confidential, as we did not want any more gatecrashers.

There was a great turnout of politicians and women. Many spoke in support. We again emphasised the categories that needed to be covered by a redress scheme.

It was decided to set up an all-party committee of deputies to brief Minister Mary Harney and report back to us at a meeting the following week in the Dáil itself. We were very pleased at this development. Sirena Campbell was there with a laptop; that threw people a bit until we found out who she was. No worries, it was okay.

"I spoke to Mary Harney today and she said the Inquiry would be reporting at the beginning of March and she will meet us then. It was a very short time so that was okay," Sirena told us. This was the first we had heard of this.

At the meeting we also received an acknowledgement of our letter of 8 November, in the form of a copy of an acknowledgement appearing to have been sent out to us on 15 November. That letter had never reached our office. Later, Sirena Campbell said in a very embarrassed way that the Minister knew that no acknowledgement had been sent and she was sorry about that.

A few women spoke at the meeting and did interviews for *Morning Ireland* and *Loose Talk*.

A short time later I got a phone call from Judge Harding Clark. "The Inquiry is going very well from our point of view," she said. "I hesitate to say that but it seems to be so."

She was getting a lot of co-operation from doctors, nurses and everyone she needed to talk to her. "Your colleague Dr O'Sullivan has been in to see us and he was a very impressive witness indeed." I said I knew he had been in but had not spoken to him since, but that the women thought him a great person.

"I need more help, more information, from Patient Focus. The names and addresses of your members and the procedures they underwent." I agreed to do my best about that but we would need the women's permission for confidentiality reasons. We got that permission easily later.

"Has Dr Neary been interviewed?" I asked her.

"Not yet, but I want to speak to him last of all, as I have certain questions to put to him," she said. She was still interviewing. Then she said, "I don't know where the idea came from that the report would be ready on 1 March. We expect to be finished interviewing, but it will take me another two to three months to write up the report."

So now we had better information to go to the meeting with the all-party Oireachtas support group in the Dáil in early February. The Ceann Comhairle, Rory O'Hanlon, also offered to meet us in his office at 6.30 p.m. before the meeting. We prepared a statement in an open letter to the Minister, stating that we had not heard from her, that now it was clear that the inquiry would not be reporting until May/June at the earliest and that she should meet us.

We were graciously received by the Ceann Comhairle in his beautiful office. He explained that he was separate from party politics. We understood. We all sat down at another magnificent table. Dr O'Hanlon listened to our arguments, put forward in the letter, for a redress board. He listened to the stories of Neary and the wounds inflicted by the doctor;

the word "mutilation" was uttered. It seemed to sink deep into the heart of a fellow doctor.

The setting up of the Patient Focus All Party Oireachtas Support Group was a very significant development. It came about as a result of our meeting between the women and local representations. These meetings were held in the Oireachtas Committee round table meeting rooms in the Millennium Building of Leinster House. Mary Wallace was elected Chair of the Group and Caoimhghín Ó Caoláin was co-ordinator.

We heard too from the *Loose Talk* programme that the Fianna Fáil parliamentary party meeting agreed to call on Minister Harney to establish a redress board to meet the needs of the women in Drogheda. The motion was put forward by Jim Glennon, the North Dublin TD. This was brilliant news. We heard that Bertie Ahern personally handed it to the Minister for Health. I rang around and told people. It gave hope.

Seamus Kirk was also supporting us. "This matter is urgent and needs to be attended to," he said. We were delighted. Another hurdle over.

The phone rang. My caller ID said "private". The woman wouldn't tell me her name. "I am afraid of a woman in Drogheda," she said. The caller with no name asked me about the missing files.

"I can't talk to people who won't identify themselves," I said. "After all, you know who I am. I need to know who you are too."

"Mary." I barely hear it.

"Mary, is it?"

338

"Yes."

"I need more than that."

"I'm afraid; I live in the area."

"I understand, but I need more than Mary. I need a surname and personal contact details. You have nothing to be afraid of. The guards are dealing with this business."

"But this person is very well in with the guards. There is this guard . . ." she said.

I stopped her. "I'd love to talk to you, Mary, but I just can't. I need details. The guards are the people to go to about the files."

"I don't know anything about where the files are or anything," she said, "but I am personally involved."

"Sorry, I can't talk to you."

"I will think about it and maybe ring back tomorrow," Mary said.

"That's fine," I said.

I rang the senior garda in charge of the Neary investigation about this call and also about recent strange emails we had been receiving about the missing files.

"This is an attempt to muddy the waters," he said, "an attempt to make you concerned about the integrity of the Gardaí."

I knew he was right and my caller never rang back.

On 11 February 2005, just as we were becoming very concerned that nothing was happening, Cathriona got a call from the Tánaiste's office with an appointment for 9 March. On 22 February, a letter arrived from Mary Harney's office, dated 9 February, acknowledging our November letter about setting up a redress board. It stated: "The Tánaiste has arranged to meet with Patient Focus on 9 March to discuss this request. Following that meeting, the Tánaiste will consider the matter in consultation with government colleagues." At last we are being told directly, we felt.

At the end of February the silent phone calls started again. Aideen answered one of them. She did not like it. I rang the gardaí again. Every time there is publicity surrounding Neary, this happened.

We should have felt we were getting places when Mary Harney spoke on local radio on the last day of February, but to be truthful we didn't, such was our battle fatigue by now. This was the first real interview in which a Minister talked about the Drogheda scandal. Such is the power of the profession and the taboo about confronting medical abuse, it still hasn't happened nationally. It happened because she was out canvassing for Sirena Campbell in the Meath by-election and a journalist essentially availed of the opportunity to doorstep her.

"The report is delayed until late April," she said, "so I will meet Patient Focus shortly. I can't make any decision about redress until Judge Harding Clark's report is available. I will explore all options. But we need to know what we are talking about. I have huge sympathy for the women, many of whose lives were destroyed. The inquiry will tell us why it went on for so long with no efforts made to change the practice."

When asked if she thought it would be helpful if Neary talked to the inquiry, she replied, "Of course it would helpful if he gives evidence. But I don't want to say anything that would jeopardise the outcome. This issue will be resolved legally."

This was an undoubted breakthrough, but we were worn out waiting for "this issue to be resolved legally".

We heard from the TDs Mary Wallace and Trevor Sargent that they had a meeting with the Minister at 3.00 p.m. on Tuesday, 8 March, the day before we were to meet her.

29

Kurtis's Case

In the week we first met the Tánaiste Mary Harney as Minister for Health, we were also supporting Kathryn Quilty through the civil case taken on behalf of her son Kurtis against the North Eastern Health Board and Michael Neary. This was a medical negligence action, as Kurtis was profoundly brain-damaged when born and his very young mother Kathryn had her womb taken out by Neary. She was barely twenty years of age.

Kurtis's case first opened in the High Court on 25 January 2005. All day the lawyers wheeled and dealed in the corridor outside Court 9. Expert witnesses from Canada and Britain waited around with the rest of us. By day's end, the junior doctor, Neary and the North Eastern Health Board had accepted liability for the damage to Kurtis at birth. No agreement was reached on damages, so a separate assessment of damages hearing had to be listed.

It was 1 March before we returned. We all collected in a room provided. Again we waited round all day. No judge was found.

"That case is listed for several weeks' hearing," I heard.

"That's awful," I said "it's purely about money; liability has been accepted. How can that take weeks?"

The next day we got a judge – Justice Herbert. For the next week Kathryn and her mother Valerie sat in court listening to the sad story of Kurtis's life, as told through his paediatrician. Cathriona, Anna and I came as support. We heard how good a mother Kathryn was to him, that she never gave the paediatrician any cause for concern, how he had experience of child protection cases but that it never arose in Kurtis's case, not even a hint. He described a happy, well-cared-for infant and later a growing child.

We heard about Kurtis's sight. Experts debated whether he was blind or not – one saying he was functionally blind and others totally disagreeing. A video with Kurtis as "star" clearly showed he was not.

Another issue revolved around whether or not Kurtis could speak. Kathryn and her mum were horrified by these arguments.

"I can speak to him. He understands me, speaks to me," his mother said quietly to me. "So can mum." Experts said he could communicate, could speak to his mother and to his granny, and they could clearly understand him. On and on it went.

The defence were seeking Kathryn's childhood medical records from Wales. It was the same barrister, Mary Irvine, who had prosecuted Neary in the Medical Council, now arguing for the other side, as barristers do. The insurance company was defending this case. The questions asked by Mary Irvine, barrister for the insurers, related to Kathryn as a mother and a person. Did she not turn up to this medical appointment or that?

"Are they saying Kurtis would be better off in a home or in foster care than with me?" Kathryn whispered to me, hands moving restlessly on the bench beside me. But professional witness after professional witness said she was a warm, attentive mother who clearly loved Kurtis, that he needed a home, needed his mother, would benefit from her care, missed her when she was not there. Kurtis needed special equipment and a house adapted to his needs.

A clinical psychologist gave evidence of Kurtis's condition, saying he was aware of his mother and was attached to her. "Kurtis is a people person," she said.

Towards the end of the questioning, Mary Irvine asked the psychologist, "Would it not be better if Kurtis had siblings?" Kathryn and her mum got very upset at this but tried not to register it. Kathryn couldn't have more children. Neary had made sure of that.

The judge said, "Surely you mean peers? We all know siblings are not possible."

The talk had moved on from residential home now to foster home. None of the experts agreed that either residential care or foster care would be best for Kurtis; full-time help for his mother was what was needed, with respite care at the weekend. This would mean he could live with Kathryn. This is what Gillian O'Connor and Michael Boylan, Kurtis's solicitors, had worked so hard for. Was Mary Irvine trying to demonstrate otherwise? Sometimes Cathriona and I tried to greet Mary Irvine, but we could never make eye contact.

On 9 March, the day we first met Mary Harney, several women came to court to support Kathryn *en route* to the

Minister. Kathryn really appreciated it. At the end of that week, the case was adjourned until 20 April.

The night before meeting Mary Harney, we met the local TDs in the room where the Joint Oireachtas Committee hearing had taken place in 2001. Mary Wallace as chair assured us, "Mary Harney is sympathetic to the women."

That was not good enough. "We've had four years of Micheál Martin's sympathy," I said. "We are worn out by sympathy; we want her to do something."

All the TDs spoke, one after the other. We told them that the judge had phoned and said she would be interviewing until the end of February and then would take two to three months to write up her report. There was no way it would be ready soon.

The TDs worried about the terms of reference of the inquiry and what damage we wanted covered by the redress. Again we mentioned all the women we wanted covered. All had strong medico-legal reports supporting their claims. Our solicitor repeated the difficulties about the missing files, the lack of indemnity as the MDU was refusing cover, and the small number of cases against another doctor.

"There were other issues in the hospital, weren't there?" the TDs asked. "The Minister is worried about this, extending redress to all of this."

Clearly the mention of redress to a politician or a civil servant causes them to see "floodgates" and think "ring-fences". If ring-fencing wasn't possible, even the most worthy calls for a redress scheme would be ignored. We restated over and over what the damage was and what the numbers were. It was as if the next answer would be different if the question was asked again. We repeated the small number of women involved but the importance of including all, not just women who had unnecessary caesarean hysterectomies.

"They don't want to open the floodgates" was the message we heard.

We met the Minister in her office in Leinster House as arranged, a very lovely set of rooms decorated in a sunny yellow with cream, coffee and chocolate-coloured carpets. The inner office too was the same colour with rich mahogany table and chairs. There were good vibes on entry. We sat around the long table, Niamh next to Mary Harney.

"You look very young," the Minister said, moved and worried by her youth.

She could give us no firm commitment at that stage except to say that no patient or doctor would be left uncovered by the MDU's default. "But once the report comes out I will act fast to resolve the matter. I accept that the idea of a redress board is the best approach and is the only idea on the table."

She looked at Niamh again just before we left. "You're so young."

All in all it was a positive meeting; brief but useful.

On 20 April we were all back again in Court 9, for another week of experts, all talking about Kurtis and Kathryn.

Kathryn took the stand on Wednesday, 27 April. Her barrister Denis McCullough took her through her tragic life. They put it all out there to be seen. She was a very powerful witness. She was frank and honest about her life and behaviour; about her love for Kurtis her son; about her hysterectomy at twenty, when she fell under Neary's knife. At the time, she did not even know what a hysterectomy was. She was just given a booklet about it, written for middle aged women and older, and that was all. Denis took her through everything, all the way to the murder of her partner, when she was also left for dead, her father's death in a fire when she was seventeen, his violence to her mother, her fosterage on her own initiative to a friend's house at the age of eleven because she didn't like her mother's new partner.

When Mary Irvine started her cross-examination, she started slowly. She talked about the equipment Kurtis might need. We were very afraid of what was to come, that it would hurt Kathryn, would be too much to bear. So I brought her and Valerie out to my house and we went for a beautiful meal that night as sustenance for what was to come.

Kathryn was not feeling well next morning and could not cope with taking the stand when she arrived at court at 10.30 a.m. She had concerns about Kurtis and his eating arrangements and toileting requirements. The residential facility where he was cared for was concerned about this too and had contacted Kathryn. Gillian, Kathryn's solicitor, phoned the social worker and Kathryn was reassured Kurtis was okay.

By noon she said she wanted to give her evidence and get it over with; she felt strong enough. The questioning was now very painful to witness. It looked to me like a deer being torn apart by a lioness, every negative aspect of Kathryn's life torn apart in forensic detail, despite the fact that she had owned up to them all. Every drink she consumed, every incident, every row, every complaint about her was raised. It went on until 4.00 p.m., with a break for lunch. She withstood it, though, explaining as best she could how broken she was, how remorseful she was for her drinking, the physical problems she had after her hysterectomy, how she loved her child, how he never suffered – she always made sure of that. When she was in trouble emotionally, she would leave Kurtis with his grannies. She'd had surgeries too, for gynaecological problems, and a breakdown.

I found all this very hard to stomach indeed. It was torture to watch, never mind experience. Kathryn was not on trial for any offence, nor was she under investigation as an unfit parent. That Thursday, the case was adjourned until Tuesday, 3 May.

Kathryn was very sad over the weekend, so we sent her flowers, enough to fill her house. We arrived early on Tuesday to the Four Courts. Kathryn was very tired but she wanted to continue. She wanted it over with; the longer this went on, the worse it would be. We heard a rumour that the claims manager from the insurers was there that morning.

Kathryn continued for another day. Her huge eyes, frail body, soft low voice, telling her story, defending herself, admitting guilt, tearful from time to time but recovering, giving as good as she got later on.

"I feel like I am on trial here for murder," she said. No one wanted to talk about her depression, about her hospital experience or her hysterectomy; about how she worried desperately that her child would die; about how she didn't feel like a woman any more after the hysterectomy; how she would never have any more children; how she wanted Kurtis with her.

The next morning, settlement talks were underway. It was after lunch before we all went back to the courtroom, to hear that a settlement had been reached. It was accepted in Court 10 before Justice de Valera. The settlement was € 3.75 million.

Afterwards, Mary Irvine hugged Kathryn and cried. "No hard feelings," the barrister said through her tears. Kathryn's face registered nothing. Her body looked stiff under the force of this embrace. Kathryn did not cry.

I believe the brutality of the legal process for traumatised patients is an abuse. A persecuted Kathryn fought for her son, her one and only child. She is a survivor. In this case it didn't work because, as Kathryn said, she was "fighting for her son". But I have to wonder, if it was herself she was fighting for, would she have had the energy and grit to keep going? She held her own, gave as good as she got, even got the upper hand in a system that was designed to break her, in an environment that overawes, by practices that humiliate.

30

Waiting for a Judge

The rest of 2005 was a time of waiting – waiting for Judge Harding Clark's report this time. We were in constant contact with the Department and with journalists. We were given many publication dates, but none of them materialised. The original timeframe estimated by Minister Martin was clearly way off the mark.

In early June, the *Sunday Tribune* reported that it was ready and would be available at the end of that month.

"I don't know where that came from," Denis O'Sullivan from the Department said when I called him, adding, "There is no date yet."

"It wasn't ready in March, now it isn't ready in June. When will it be ready?" I asked. Denis didn't know.

Later we learnt, via the medical press, that Neary was co-operating with the inquiry. It was apparent that the inquiry was ongoing despite our earlier reassurances it would be completed by March.

But there were small victories too. Mary Harney made the very important decision to let the women have an advance viewing of the report. We raised this in a letter and follow-up parliamentary question from Deputy Fergus O'Dowd. Without this back-up strategy, we doubted if the Minister would see our letter asking to let us see the report before it was published.

We went to meet the Patient Focus Oireachtas Support Group on a very beautiful evening in June to discuss the details of how this might happen and to press again for redress, and to reiterate the numbers and categories of damage involved, of the twenty-five women who would not fit neatly into a rigid scheme confined to caesarean hysterectomies. We raised the issue of a Dáil debate once the report was out too.

A medical journalist also spoke to the nuns' PR company, Gibney Public Relations. "I phoned the headquarters of the Medical Missionaries of Mary in Booterstown and was referred to Gibney PR. The response I received there was a threefold 'no comment'," he told us. The women felt the limited engagement by the nuns was a scandal in itself.

Fidelma contacted the Medical Missionaries of Mary to ask them to meet us.

"I will pass it on to the nuns," said the woman who answered the phone.

A Sister Isobel returned her call. "The nuns feel it would be inappropriate to meet the women before the report comes out."

"When the report comes out will you meet us?"

"I would have to get back to the nuns with that."

At the end of June there was a public reference to Drogheda by the Minister for Health at an HSE conference on "People Matter – Complaints Matter". Cathriona and I were in attendance. Mary Harney spoke of how important complaints were – indeed, how valuable they were. She spoke of being at a recent conference in Geneva where Sir Liam Donaldson talked of medical negligence. She quoted him as saying: "In America you have a one in 3,000,000 chance of dying in an aeroplane crash and a one in 300 chance of dying as a result of medical negligence." She spoke of the importance of the forthcoming report into Drogheda and the likelihood that malpractice continued for so long because there was nowhere to complain. We felt she was talking directly to us.

In early July, I spoke to Jim Reilly. "Any news about the report?" I asked. "Could it be delayed till the end of this month?"

"Yes," he said. "It looks like Neary has visited them in Bow Street."

"He's gone to the inquiry?" I asked.

"That is what I am hearing, but it has not been confirmed."

"Are you worried about the final report in any way?" I asked.

"No, not at all," he said, "but I hope they can see through him. He will probably blame everyone else."

Driving along the motorway later, I started thinking of Neary being interviewed by the judge. A tiny woman judge and a large bulky man. I imagined him weaving stories as he did in the High Court.

On 11 July, local radio rang. "We have a pre-recorded interview with Bertie Ahern on the Neary scandal. Do you want to hear it?"

I was stripping wallpaper at time, but of course I wanted to hear the Taoiseach. They arranged to put me online to listen as they broadcast the interview. At last Bertie would say something in public, and about time too, I thought.

When asked about the report of the inquiry and what he had to say to the women concerned, Bertie said that it was a very worrying case and the government had discussed it many times. He said the report was due to be published very soon, maybe even before the holidays, "So until then we can't comment on its content. After receiving it and considering it, we look forward to commenting." He could, he said, assure us that "the government will not be found wanting". We took this as a promise of appropriate redress for damaged women.

That was the first time the Taoiseach had spoken in public about the issue.

By August there was still no news of the report. A phone call to the Department told me that it would not be ready now until September at least. The Minister was on holidays, and all departments, even PR people, would have to see it, not to mind those directly affected by it. All in all, conversations got awkward with the Department. My feeling was that they had no good news so they didn't want to give any.

Early in the month too, we heard from *The Irish Times* that that no criminal charges were possible in relation to the missing files. This came as no great surprise as the gardaí had found none of the original files.

The women kept busy during these months of waiting for the inquiry report. Its effect on them was different. They created a memory board. We were bearing witness again, praying if you like. Women sent us poems, photos, mementos. We laid them out on a table. These were amazingly moving. It took me all my time to cope sometimes. Kathryn sent in a matinée coat and babygro. Noeleen, Teresa, Alma, a very quiet and private woman, among others looked out from photos and held babies that were now grown. They wore flares and their men had long hair. They looked like Niamh, so young were they in these pictures from the '70s and '80s. There were many Niamhs and Kathryns over the twenty-four years of Neary's practice.

For me it was an altar. Cathriona said, "Birthdays are like anniversaries of sorts." So too were first smiles, first tooth, first step, first day at school, college and so on. All anniversaries of sorts. Our altar acted as a sort of poultice too. But mostly they were memories laid out as treasures. A matinée coat or baby hat became holy as we celebrated the infant they warmed. It was as if the women had washed and ironed baby things, folded and scented them, wrapping them in tissue in a secret drawer to be looked at and honoured from time to time when they needed to.

By September the women were restless for news of the report. I rang Denis O'Sullivan, worried.

"Will you talk to the judge this evening?" he asked when he rang back later.

"Yes, of course."

"The delay is because it's a private inquiry. Everyone has to be given a right of reply to adverse findings made against them."

Judge Harding Clark called that evening. She introduced herself as Maureen Clark. She wanted to fill us in on dates and times. "I would like nothing better than to sit down with the women at this stage and show them the report. But I am not allowed to," she told me. There was genuine regret in her voice. She confirmed that the report was written and had to be circulated to certain people. I said the women were annoyed that Neary would see it before them.

In this way the heat was taken out of the waiting.

Cathriona, Maura and three women from Louth went to visit Dermot Ahern, the Minister for Foreign Affairs, looking for his support. This meeting did not go well. The women felt that he had not been that supportive; it came across as lukewarm to them at best. They were particularly upset because he is a local Minister.

I emailed Judge Harding Clark at the beginning of December asking for an update. She replied that the report was ready but legal niceties were still being tidied up. Later we spoke on the phone. "I am going to recommend that women with missing files get a substantial lump sum," she said. In relation to a redress board, she said that legally she couldn't recommend one, as the state had no liability since the Lourdes was a private hospital.

I told her that the Department of Health was still leading us to believe that a redress board would be announced when the report was published. This was also the view of the local TDs. "It would be a disaster for the women if there was no redress," I said.

"I just get that impression talking to Finance," she said. "I was looking for a little more funding; I am now without any staff too, which makes this very difficult for me."

"I can imagine," I said.

"The difficulty is," she said, "that I believe there is a tightening of the purse strings, and people are fearful of redress."

Cans of worms, floodgates and ring-fencing shouted out at me as she said this.

The Christmas deadline passed but Judge Harding Clark kept in touch to update us on likely finishing dates. We arranged a meeting with the women for 19 January 2006 to pass on this information.

In early January RTÉ approached us again about making another programme for screening the night the report come out. We arranged for the programme makers to come to our meeting in the Boyne Valley. This time we had no difficulty getting people to talk on camera. I was amazed at the recovery.

The meeting was very positive and upbeat. Some of the women decided to make criminal complaints about their medical care by Neary. They felt the level of negligence involved amounted to criminal negligence. A number of women who had caesarean hysterectomies were interviewed in great detail by Gardaí. Neary himself was interviewed. A file was prepared for the Director of Public Prosecutions. However the DPP decided there was insufficient evidence of intent to charge Neary with a criminal offence.

Susan Mitchell wrote an article, "A System in Need of Treatment", in the *Sunday Business Post* on 15 January 2006:

356

The Irish Hospital Consultants' Association believes Ireland's compensation culture, fuelled by ambulance-chasing solicitors, is largely to blame for Ireland's allegedly high rates of litigiousness. Finbarr Fitzpatrick, general secretary of the Irish Hospital Consultants' Association, said radical action was needed. Fitzpatrick said the level of claims remained a huge concern.

He said, "Irish consultants are four times as likely to be sued as British consultants." Fitzpatrick said court awards were significantly higher in Ireland than in most other countries. This, he said, has resulted in exorbitant insurance costs for consultants, particularly those working in obstetric and gynaecology, who suffer the bulk of claims.

The women who read this were deeply offended. Three years before, they had heard Finbarr Fitzpatrick express a similar view in Mike Milotte's *Bad Medicine*, a *Prime Time* special investigation on the extent of medical errors in Ireland, screened on 15 December 2003. Speaking about medical negligence claims and on behalf of the IHCA, he had said, "We totally accept . . . that there are people who have a just case and are deserving of redress, but I think it would be incorrect to assume that the compensation culture which has been highlighted with regard to business and industry and the problems it has created for a lot of small industries with regard to insurance does not necessarily apply in the world of health."

The women felt that nothing could be further from the truth in relation to the solicitors they used. They felt too that they were being criticised for taking legal action, a route they felt morally obliged to travel.

On 23 January, RTÉ News revealed that the same Finbarr Fitzpatrick was at the meeting with Neary and the health board in October 1998. He would have been aware of the serious allegation against Neary. Later, he would have known Neary had been found guilty by the Medical Council. Also, he had sourced the three doctors who gave Neary's practice a clean bill of health, supporting the doctor against the health board when they tried to remove Neary from the hospital in the weeks after the midwives voiced their complaints in October 1998.

On 26 January, Judge Harding Clark rang. "The report is finished," she told me, "and it is to be delivered to the Minister tomorrow. The appointment is for 4.00 p.m." She wanted feedback from the women and said she hoped the report was fair. I thanked her for doing it. It was expected to be placed before cabinet the following Tuesday, 31 January.

"That's Seamus's birthday; he will be ten on Tuesday," Cathriona said when I told her. The end of January was always a difficult period for several of the women. In January 1996, Neary performed six caesarean hysterectomies.

At that time too we heard from Niamh that the MDU had withdrawn from her case. It was gone off record. They would not insure Neary for the damage he had caused her.

Then the missing files delayed everything again. At their meeting, the judge revealed to Minister Harney that, in the last day or so, more information had come her way and she had to look into it.

Denis O'Sullivan contacted me about the meeting, and summarised the report. The judge's verdict was that the system let down the doctor and the doctor let down the patients. No sense of badness. It was the culture of the hospital, the ethos of the nuns. No one told, no one knew, the extent of caesarean hysterectomies in the hospital, he explained. This turned out to be a very accurate summary of the report.

At the conversation's end, Denis told me, "The report will not be put to cabinet now for two more weeks. I don't know what the rush is anyway. Particularly because it raises the spectre of redress."

"An interesting Freudian slip," I said.

"What do you mean?" he asked, genuinely not knowing.

"Redress as a spectre?"

"Oh, you know what I mean," he said.

"I do." Cans of worms, floodgates, ring-fences!

So, a Department of Health official was telling us that the removal of healthy organs from healthy young women was a culture. Was he saying we had a corrupt culture of care in one of our hospitals? I slowly realised how damning this was of the medical system – a hospital and a doctor out of control; patients at the mercy of bent and powerful ideologies, so powerful no one even questioned it. It was very scary. Doctors' pathologies can be a danger to all. Later, when I told Cathriona, she said, "This is institutional abuse; it's just like a cult." She was right.

On the day I spoke to Denis, the Minister was in Dundalk where she was interviewed by LMFM. She was asked about the report. She indicated that the report would not be going to Cabinet the following Tuesday. We were also worried by the Minister's mention of redress for the women whose files are missing, but no more.

Most of the women and their families believed that in a decent country this matter would have been in the criminal courts long ago. But here in Ireland, because of power and position, it was not so. Several women wanted to make complaints to the Gardaí, alleging criminal negligence and assault by Michael Neary when he removed their womb. Patient Focus wrote to the Commissioner asking him to allow the National Bureau of Criminal Investigation to conduct any inquiry. The women knew these gardaí from the missing files investigation and had found them professional and sensitive.

I got a call from a journalist after this. "Are you not afraid of being charged with 'malicious prosecution'?"

"How could I be?" I said. "I can't prosecute anyone. It is the DPP who decides that, not me. I won't be making any complaints about Neary. The women in our group have always told the facts as they are. Told the truth. So have   I."

"Neary will do anything to defend himself," the journalist said.

"I have no doubt about that," I said, "but I have done nothing wrong."

I reiterated that it was the women who would make statements, the Gardaí who would investigate them and the DPP who would decide matters after that. I stated clearly that I deeply resented the implication in the question. The journalist apologised.

So, the month ended with us still waiting, but knowing there was a cultural corruption at the heart of the Lourdes hospital.

In the run-up to the publication of the report, we reflected on the pieces of information we had been given about its contents. In Drogheda, the practice of caring had become self-serving. It became a need to be wonderful, a need to save lives that were not at risk, a need to save women who wanted babies from pregnancy. It was expressed as "solving their family planning problems" before they had that family, before they had any children in some cases.

Neary, a very nice man and doctor, mutilated a large number of women. He did not believe he had done anything wrong. In the unit, seemingly no one noticed. It was normal. The abnormal became normalised, the irrational was rationalised. How did this happen?

It is, I think, about how so-called caring relationships go wrong, because of an imbalance of power between the carer and the cared-for. Because the dominant culture is created by those caring, terrible things can happen. The "care" can be diverted into filling the needs of the care-giver, rather than the cared-for. It is as if the care-giver owns the cared-for. And isn't that potential pathology built into the doctor–patient relationship when it is hard to change doctors, when it is next to impossible to get a second opinion? When one doctor will not see another doctor's patients, especially in private medicine?

But not only did the internal culture within the Lourdes favour Neary over patients; so too did the external one. Three eminent doctors and their union's Secretary General defended his practices. The doctor came first in all these occasions.

Medical ethics should not be the preserve of doctors

alone. There needs to be constant balancing of modes of behaviour, and thought and belief systems. In Drogheda, a doctor was out of line, a unit was out of line, other issues were placed before the interests of patients and patients were routinely humiliated and damaged.

On Monday, Tuesday and Wednesday of the week commencing 20 February, we rang the Department for news. We finally discovered that publication would be on Tuesday, 28 February. With that settled, we started to ask when we were going to get an advance copy. There were difficulties about us getting an advance copy. There was also an indication that publication might be further delayed.

"I can't go back to the women again and say it is off for another week," I said, asking for help. Denis talked about his fear of leaks. "We will not leak the report," I said.

On the Friday morning I was told that the Tánaiste was in Vienna for an EU meeting. The implication was that we could not get an advance copy without the Minister's agreement, and she wasn't contactable. We rang Deputy Jim Glennon, who was a passionate supporter. He wanted to help. He said it was essential the women received an advance copy. Later Denis rang to say that the Tánaiste was on her way back to Dublin, and that the report could be released to us that afternoon.

Late in the afternoon, I went to the Department to get the report. "No leaks, make sure," Denis said as he handed me a copy of the report in the foyer of Hawkins House.

"Any chance of a copy for all the women?" I said.

"That's impossible. It would be an insult to the

Oireachtas if that happened." I asked him to run that past me again; he repeated it.

I was so worn out with the effort needed to get the report that I couldn't look at it that night. I put it safely away in my hall table, unopened. I was able to tell journalists who phoned that the Minister had kept her word, that we had an advance copy. There was no chance I would give them any information on its contents. I had to tell the women first.

Next day I opened the report. We gathered the committee together, called Colm and met in the office. Colm prepared a summary over the weekend and we set about phoning each and every woman in the group between the five of us. The first impressions were good but we needed to have a meeting on the Monday night before it went to Cabinet on Tuesday and was published.

But on Sunday, it was all over the *Sunday Tribune*. We emailed the journalist who wrote the story to complain. He never replied.

On Monday morning Denis O'Sullivan called to say he did not know where the leak came from, but it was just one chapter, a draft chapter, not the whole report. He reiterated about us not leaking. I felt extremely bothered. I was not going to leak; we had to have a meeting with our women. Why would I leak?

The meeting that night was a great one. Everyone was relieved when we told them that the story was good enough.

Part 5

Some Answers

31

Report of The Lourdes Hospital Inquiry

Judge Harding Clark's report made some very important findings from the women's point of view.

Firstly, she found that the rate of peripartum hysterectomy at the unit from 1974 to 1998 was "truly shocking". She discovered that 188 such operations were carried out in the unit as a whole and, of those, 129 were carried out by Dr Neary over twenty-five years. Of concern too was the youth of his patients and the low number of children they had before hysterectomy. Twenty-five hysterectomies involved women having their first child. Included in this figure were two women whose babies died and so were without children of their own. Included also were two nineteen-year-olds and two twenty-year-olds. Twenty-six women were having their second baby at the time of hysterectomy and of the remaining cases, twenty-six mothers had three children. A crude statistic was that forty per cent of Dr Neary's patients were having their first or second baby.

The several midwives who told of their concerns from about 1996 were concerned at the younger age and low parity of Dr Neary's patients. The Matron was worried about Dr Neary's rising caesarean hysterectomy rate. But Judge Harding Clark concluded that no one made a formal complaint and no one questioned openly. She said:

"Few complained or questioned:

- *not the patients, their partners nor their families*

- *not the obstetricians who worked in the Maternity Unit and who knew of the operations carried out*

- *not the junior doctors nor the post membership registrars*

- *not the anaesthetists, who received the patient, administered the anaesthesia, wrote up the operation notes and spoke to each patient in the recovery room and were always present at the operations*

- *not the surgical nurses, who were frequently midwives, and always women, who handed the hysterectomy clamps to the surgeons and counted the swabs*

- *not the midwives who cared for the women after their operations and who recorded each day the women stayed in the post natal ward and the fact that they had had a peripartum hysterectomy*

- *not the pathologists and technicians who received the wombs and specimens from the maternity theatre, who dissected, examined and reported*

- *not the Matrons who made ward rounds and who contacted the public health nurses*

- *not the Sisters of the Medical Missionaries of Mary who owned the hospital and employed the obstetricians*

- *not one of the various GPs whose patients attended the IMTH [International Missionary Teaching Hospital] and underwent caesarean hysterectomy*

- *not any of the parties who read the maternity hospital's biennial reports in the years when it was published.*

Judge Harding Clark noted too that the Royal College of Obstetricians and Gynaecologists inspected the Maternity Unit in 1987 and 1992 and found it to be suitable for training obstetric registrars. Their approval was lukewarm and suggestions were made but never followed up. An Bord Altranais too made suggestions about family planning and midwife training, but nothing happened.

She concluded that no person or institution raised any issues until October 1998, when two experienced midwives sought the health board solicitor's advice on serious concerns which one of the midwives had about Dr Neary's practices.

Judge Harding Clark's examination of the missing records issue was forensic and a very disturbing aspect of the Dr Neary saga. The inquiry was satisfied *"that a person or persons unidentified, who had knowledge of where records were stored and who had easy access to those records, was responsible for a deliberate, careful and systematic removal of key historical records, together with master cards and patient charts. Three alterations to the maternity theatre register detected by the Inquiry appear to be made in the same hand and apparently were made after complaints were made against Dr Neary. Most of the missing records refer to Dr Neary's patients. Someone with a misplaced sense of loyalty to Dr Neary or the unit is probably responsible."*

Judge Harding Clark said that the story of Dr Neary's fall from grace was one of enormous tragedy, for the hospital, for the staff, and especially for the women who entered the hospital to face the joy of a new baby and who returned home to recuperate from a hysterectomy. She stated: *"This is not a simple story of an evil man or a bad doctor, nor is it a story of wholesale suppression of facts . . . There was no attempt to hide the procedures or pretend they were something else . . . Neither is it the story of a surgeon with poor surgical skills or a doctor deficient in academic excellence . . . His trainers speak very highly of him . . . It is the story of a doctor who at critical points during his training was inadequately supervised. It is the story of a doctor with a deep fault line, which was recognised early but never corrected."*

Judge Harding Clark wrote about the culture of the hospital, of a maternity unit caught in a time warp. Every hospital since the 1970s saw a fall in its rate of hysterectomy following caesarean section. Every hospital in the state, that is, except the Lourdes. She described a rigid hierarchical structure at the unit, based on division of tasks, everyone knowing their place, with no possibility of questioning by subservient nurses. Loyalty also developed because of the lack of movement of staff. Non-national doctors were reluctant to question consultants because they depended on them for references, but some Irish junior doctors believed Dr Neary suffered from a personality disorder.

The lack of sterilisation too served to muddy the waters as to the reasons for hysterectomy, with some people believing that the hysterectomies were hidden sterilisations.

Power in the hospital was difficult to locate, with consultants believing it rested with the management and management believing it rested with consultants.

Judge Harding Clark described a doctor who probably had a phobic reaction to blood and at the same time practised a technique of swabbing, dabbing and poking at small bleeding points and at the uterus, which probably encouraged bleeding. She never-theless decided that there was probably a personality defect at play, which prevented a competent surgeon from appreciating the heartache of a hysterectomy to a woman.

The inquiry confirmed a belief that it was very difficult for management to remove Dr Neary from practice at the hospital. The process started in October 1998 after two midwives reported their concern that Dr Neary was carrying out an unduly large number of caesarean hysterectomies at the unit where they worked.

Dr Neary was asked to take administrative leave for two weeks in order that the allegations could be investigated. At the end of this period, Dr Neary wanted to return to work. But Dr Ambrose McLoughlin, the Assistant CEO of the Health Board, had serious and reasonable misgivings about this. He wanted Dr Neary's return to be subject to a peer review of his caesarean hysterectomy rate between 1996 and 1998 and an audit by the Institute of Obstetricians and Gynaecologists of Ireland.

Dr Neary initially consented to this but later argued

through his representatives that this would be so damaging to him that civil damages would not be sufficient remedy. Dr Neary's advisors then obtained copy files of the seventeen cases of caesarean hysterectomy performed in the period 1996–1998. He had these cases reviewed by three established, eminent and practising consultant colleagues in Dublin.

The three obstetricians met together with Dr Neary and considered the files in turn. At all stages they accepted the explanations provided by Dr Neary. Eight of the seventeen cases they were asked to review were excluded because Dr Neary informed them that these were consent hysterectomies – necessitated because of the prohibition in the hospital of tubal ligations.

The three doctors produced two reports. Two of the obstetricians concluded:

> *Having reviewed the case notes we are of the opinion that all of the nine cases reviewed can be justified in the prevailing situation . . . We find no evidence of questionable clinical judgement, poor operative ability or faulty decision making. Quite the contrary, we find that Dr Neary, in the exercise of his clinical judgement, has under difficult circumstances probably saved the lives of several mothers . . . On the evidence presented we find no grounds to suspend Dr Neary or to place any restrictions on his practice (public or private).*

The third obstetrician reported as follows:

> *I have scrutinised photocopies of the notes presented to me of the nine patients who underwent emergency*

hysterectomy in the three years 1996 to 1998 at the practice of Dr Michael Neary in Drogheda. Seven of these patients had intraoperative haemorrhage and two had a post-partum hysterectomy ... which had not responded to appropriate therapy. Dr Neary was called in to a further five cases during the three years in question to help a colleague. Dr Neary's undoubted reputation at management of postpartum haemorrhage was in my opinion life saving in these cases. From the data provided by Dr Neary his rate of caesarean hysterectomy is not dramatically different from that of his colleagues.

It is my conclusion that Dr Neary has no case to answer concerning his management of any of the patients in question. . . .

It is my firm conclusion that Dr Neary should continue to work in Our Lady of Lourdes Hospital pending any formal investigation. It would be wrong to put restrictions on his practice and it is my view that the mothers of the North Eastern Health Board are fortunate in having the service of such an experienced and caring obstetrician.

Judge Harding Clark's conclusion was that Dr Neary was thus considered "to present no danger to patients".

On receipt of these reports, the health board went abroad to seek the opinion of a British obstetrician, Dr Michael Maresh, a consultant in St Mary's Hospital, Manchester, on the same nine cases reviewed in Dublin. In his report Dr Maresh wrote:

From the information supplied I have major concerns about Dr Neary continuing to practise currently as a consultant obstetrician. His clinical judgement appears to be significantly impaired and women appear to be being put at risk. Although my concerns relate mainly to his excessive use of hysterectomy post-delivery I do have concerns of other aspects of his management of patients. In addition to his clinical judgement I have concerns about his skills at caesarean section currently if there are complications. Finally, Dr Neary's perception of events appears impaired.

Tragically many of these women who were deprived of having children in future were young. Three were having their first baby. One of the three lost her baby (through no fault of Dr Neary) and so now will never have children of her own.

Having considered the Maresh report, the CEO invoked Appendix IV of the Consultants' Contract and instructed Dr Neary to take immediate administrative leave with effect from 11 December 1998.

The three Dublin-based doctors and the solicitor involved in their reports attended for interview at the inquiry and explained to Judge Harding Clark that their limited report was prepared on a confidential basis to enable Dr Neary to continue working pending the outcome of the review of his practice by the Institute. Commenting on this, Judge Harding Clark says:

The inquiry accepts that permitting Dr Neary to work pending the review by the Institute of Obstetricians and Gynaecologists well have been the intention of his union advisors and his three colleagues in presenting their report. The report may have been prepared for limited viewing but the language, which is not qualified, is regrettable. I believe that the three obstetricians involved have had serious regrets for their parts in producing these reports, which were motivated by compassion and collegiality. They ought to have been alarmed that one obstetrician carried out seventeen caesarean hysterectomies in three years in a middle-sized maternity unit, notwithstanding the lack of tubal ligations, a vascular surgeon or the use of prostaglandins.

On 14 December 1998, full details of the nine cases reviewed by Dr Maresh were published in *The Irish Times*. The Medical Council became involved after the newspaper reported. They wrote to the NEHB requesting details. The board forwarded documentation to them in January 1999 and the name of Michael Neary was temporarily removed from the Medical Register by the High Court on 5 February, with effect from 17 February. They decided that a *prima facie* case existed for the holding of a fitness to practise inquiry.

32

Aftermath of the Report

On publication day many women and their men came to town – everyone who had ever met a politician and lots more. They packed Buswell's Hotel from 2.00 p.m., awaiting the Lourdes Hospital Report. After the cabinet meeting, An Tánaiste published the report at a press conference in Government Buildings. Deputy Mary Wallace arranged for the women to gain entry. Without fuss or clamour, they infiltrated Government Buildings and became the story. I stayed behind in the hotel and felt like a proud mother watching her confident brood fly. I got a bouquet of flowers too from Caitlin. What more could I ask for?

Many TDs from the Patient Focus Oireachtas Support Group attended to support the women once again. Mary Harney said at that time that redress was no longer an issue. From that we took that it would happen. The women took the lead in the evening news as they were filmed collecting their copies of the report.

That morning on national radio, RTÉ's *Morning Ireland*, Dr John Hillery, now President of the Medical Council, was interviewed by Áine Lawlor. Responding to the culture explanation and the need to go abroad to obtain a properly independent medical opinion, Dr Hillery said, "I listened to the stories told by the ladies who came to our [the Medical Council's] inquiry and one can only be horrified at what happened to them. I don't think culture is an excuse. I don't accept it as an explanation for what happened myself. Implicit in our training is respect for the patient. Our ethical guide says doctors have a responsibility to our patients and to the profession, and the only responsibility to the profession is to ensure patients are looked after. It is shocking that it went on for so long. People have questions to answer. We need to review the report and see what can be done."

RTÉ's *Prime Time* that night was about the events that made the report necessary. I met John Hillery in hospitality as we waited to be interviewed. He spoke of his respect for the women and for what they had done. He repeated his view that this was not only about culture. It was also about personality issues. He worried about the women and how they were now. The psychiatrist who had met the women in Lynn House so many years before said that legal change must take place before we could be sure this would not happen again. I had huge respect for this man. Clearly he found himself in a very painful place during the Medical Council inquiry.

On the programme, Dr Hillery said too that he didn't believe culture was at the root of this particular issue. "We must examine our culture," he said, referring to the profession, "and see how it is putting barriers between ourselves and patients and deal with that."

On behalf of the women, I was able to welcome the report and for the first time I was able to publicly commend officials in the NEHB for obtaining the report from the foreign expert. I also asked what would have happened to "Ann", the hero of the story, the midwife who told what was happening, had officials not supported her. I had waited a long time to be able to say this.

In the car going home from RTÉ, I got another call from Jim Glennon. "I watched the programme with the Tánaiste," he said and could say that we would be getting a redress package the next day when we met her. I rang Colm, who was exhausted, and texted Fidelma and Cathriona to tell them the news.

Our meeting with the Tánaiste and Minister for Health, Mary Harney, was extraordinary. I lost count of how many turned up to meet her. All twelve or fifteen of us were individually welcomed by the Minister standing at the door of her inner office. She shook hands with each woman and man. Seats were found for everyone. I introduced people by name and then everyone gave a little summary of their experiences in the maternity and gynaecology unit of Drogheda.

The meeting lasted an hour. Philip was "a mighty man", Mary Harney said to him as he told, in heart-rending detail, of the truly terrible experiences of his family in the Lourdes. We emphasised the breadth of damage at the hospital. It was not just caesarean hysterectomies, it was gynaecological too, as well as the babies' deaths. And yes, we were happy to have Judge Harding Clark appointed to recommend an appropriate package of redress. Every woman in the group would receive a copy of the report too.

"Do you go with the blood phobia explanation?" she asked as we prepared to leave.

"No," said Cathriona, as did others.

"I have a fear of cats so I don't keep them. If you have a fear of blood you don't go into obstetrics," said the Minister.

In the large entrance hall of Leinster House, as we stood around preparing to meet the waiting media, we saw Senator Ger Feeney, a member of the Medical Council and the Fitness to Practise committee during the Neary inquiry. She recognised us and came over. "I will never forget those hearings. Myself, I often wonder how ye kept going. I will never forget the nineteen-year-old girl with her lovely husband who gave evidence. I always remember I was having my baby in the north-west at the same time as she was having hers in the north-east under Neary in 1986," she said.

"Thank you for that. I will tell her," I replied.

The media scrum was waiting for us. Pinned to the railings of Leinster House, we told them we were very positive about the meeting; all damaged women would receive redress, we believed, including those whose babies had died and all other damaged women at the units.

Back at the office and at home, the phones were hopping like mad. Loads of new people. Tony got in touch too after *Prime Time*. Still callers to local radio spoke of the terrible effect this had on the man responsible.

The women were wonderful but it was taking its toll. Many cried when they got home. Some worried too about the reaction of the local community to them. They were still broken-hearted. But vindicated.

The Taoiseach Bertie Ahern apologised to the women during the Dáil debate that followed. "I also express my deepest regret and apologies to these women and their families for what happened. On behalf of the government we are very sorry and deeply regret what happened . . . We are all equally appalled."

Deputy Pat Rabbitte made another point during that debate: "Three obstetricians in Dublin found his conduct was flawless. That seems mind-boggling to the average citizen."

The Taoiseach replied, "As the Deputy has said, they gave a clean bill of health both to the individual and to the unit. The deputy has used his own terms for that and I will not disagree. I cannot understand that either. This raises issues for the Medical Council, which it accepts. The Minister for Health and Children has raised the issues with the Council . . . It also raises issues for the College of Obstetrics because three of its senior members examined the cases and procedures and believed that Dr Neary was fine."

The Irish Times in an article written by Eithne Donnellan named the same three men the following day: This was the second time a national paper named them.

The three Dublin-based obstetricians who conducted the review of the work of Dr Michael Neary after initial concerns were raised about his high rate of hysterectomy and found he had no case to answer have had some serious regrets, according to the Lourdes Hospital Inquiry Report. The three obstetricians are not named in the Report but The Irish Times *understands they are Professor Walter Prendiville, consultant obstetrician and gynaecologist at the Coombe Women's Hospital; Dr John Murphy, consultant obstetrician at the National Maternity Hospital, Holles St; and Dr Bernard Stuart of the Coombe Women's Hospital.*

And then came another apology, this time from the Lourdes Hospital Medical Board. In early March 2006, this letter appeared in several local and national papers:

Dear Sir,
On behalf of the current Medical Board in Our Lady of Lourdes Hospital we would like to extend a sincere and heartfelt apology to all of the women and their families affected by this tragedy. This should not have happened and should not have continued for such a long time. We would like to thank Judge Harding Clark and all her team for their courtesy, kindness and professionalism in its production. In particular we would like to acknowledge the members of Patient Focus and their spokesperson Sheila O'Connor for the courage, persistence and dignity they have shown throughout this process.

Yours sincerely
Dr Alf Nicholson,
Chairperson of the Medical Board
Dr Dominic O'Brannagain, Deputy
Chairperson of the Medical Board

Dr Shane Higgins, Lead Clinician, Dept of
Obstetrics and Gynaecology
Dr Seosamh Ó Coigligh, Deputy Lead Clinician,
Dept of Obstetrics and Gynaecology

This apology was very well received by the women and their families. However, I felt it was a pity that there was no mention of the midwife Ann, who broke these terrible concerns to the Health Board's legal advisor, or of the managers in the NEHB, Dr Ambrose McLoughlin and Mr Jim Reilly, who showed exceptional courage and dedication to helping the women discover the truth.

33

Spectre of Redress

Fifteen months later, on 18 April 2007, the Minister for Health announced the redress scheme for Dr Neary's former patients. At the top table in Government Buildings on that occasion, Minister Dermot Ahern accompanied her.

This scheme arose directly from the findings of the inquiry. The Minister acknowledged the long and difficult road travelled by the women and apologised again for what had happened to them and their families in Our Lady of Lourdes Hospital. She announced too that the redress board would be chaired by Judge Harding Clark.

The redress scheme referred to former patients of Dr Neary who underwent medically unwarranted obstetric hysterectomies at Our Lady of Lourdes Hospital during the period 1974 to 1998. The scheme also extended to cover women who underwent a medically unwarranted bilateral oophorectomy (removal of both ovaries or a single remaining ovary) while under the age of forty years. Judge Harding

Clark advised that 172 former patients of Dr Neary fell within the scope of the scheme, 122 who underwent an obstetric hysterectomy and fifty who underwent a bilateral oophorectomy under the age of forty years.

The level of award ranged from €60,000 to €260,000 in the cases of obstetric hysterectomy and €80,000 to €340,000 in the cases of bilateral oophorectomy. These were ex-gratia payments provided for by government and paid from the Department of Health and Children's budget. It is not underpinned by specific legislation and is therefore not a statutory right. A points scheme was devised based on age, procedure and number of children.

Two major issues arose for the women as a result of this announcement. One was the shock at the large number of women who had undergone bilateral oophorectomy. Furthermore, there were a number of exclusions from the scheme. In particular, the seven women mentioned specifically by name by the Minister, at the meeting prior to the announcement of the scheme, have not as yet received redress. This is despite our understanding of the political promises we received that day that these cases would be catered for by the State Claims Agency on a similar basis as the Redress Scheme.

Approximately thirty-five women with strong medical reports testifying to neglectful care have still to receive justice. These include the women over forty whose gynaecological surgery was unnecessary or negligent. In addition, it also includes the women whose babies died in very worrying circumstances at the unit.

Mary Harney acknowledged the horror experienced by the young women who had both ovaries removed unnecessarily by Neary. She included them, on the advice of Judge Harding Clark, in the redress scheme. We had always known of their existence and indeed their suffering, because a number of them were members of our group from the very beginning. Their grief was enormous, their feelings of assault overwhelming, their ability to have children gone forever, plunged unnecessarily into the menopause at a young age by a very dodgy doctor. How could it not be so!

We spoke of them over and over again to Judge Harding Clark as we "negotiated" the appropriate scope of the redress scheme, describing the effect it had on them. We knew they understated things when one woman, speaking for others, said: "I felt like an old woman in my twenties. I had no idea when I went into hospital he was going to do this. This affected by ability to form relationships with men. I have avoided intimacy because of it, afraid that no one would want me."

We did not know there were fifty women who were statistically likely to have been operated on unnecessarily. Judge Harding Clark never gave us the slightest inkling of these huge numbers. Over and over again we raised the need to acknowledge the wrong done to individual named women, totally unaware that the numbers were so high. Of course, we always knew there were more damaged women but in our worst moments we never imagined fifty or more. We always believed in Judge Harding Clark's concern about them but we always felt we had to fight tooth-and-nail to establish their violation. We spent months at it, worried incessantly about them, aware we could not agree to any scheme that did not include them, despite what we thought were the small numbers involved.

Their inclusion in the redress scheme, allied to the short time-frame for receipt of applications, necessitated that we ask the network manager in the HSE North East to write to the women and inform them of the possibility that their surgery was unnecessary, offer them counselling and a medical opinion on the matter, to establish if they qualified for the redress scheme. This proved very difficult. The HSE was not jumping to help. At first they refused to write to the women. We were told at a meeting by a senior HSE official in the North East area that "the HSE has no legal duty to tell women they may have been damaged".

To say we were gobsmacked is an understatement. Had nothing changed? Had they learnt nothing? This reinforced our anxiety that if Neary had happened in any other area of the country with different people in charge, we might never have heard about him and his trail of destruction. He would have won at the first hurdle and the two midwives would have been thrown to the lions. We had to go public and look for the women to contact us, appeal for them to contact us on national and local radio and newspapers. We had to go public to force the HSE to act. At last, about three weeks before the deadline of 12 August for receipt of applications, the HSE relented. The women were formally contacted by letter.

We also asked Dr Clements and Dr Porter to come to Ireland to see these women and provide them with opinions as to the need for their surgery. They agreed immediately. We set appointments for the women and asked the doctors to provide a general report for us on their findings. This is what they said:

From 14 to 17 August, Richard Porter and Roger Clements saw sixty-two women complaining about the treatment they received at the hands of Dr Michael Neary at Our Lady of Lourdes Hospital,

Drogheda. Of the sixty-two we saw, we concluded that thirty-nine had valid cases for compensation because of incompetent care at the hands of Dr Neary; two other cases were uncertain because of lack of notes but we thought probably deserved compensation. Twenty-one of the women did not, in our opinion, have a case for compensation.

The doctors identified a number of themes in relation to the unnecessary surgery:

Removal of Both Ovaries
Just as in the cases of caesarean hysterectomies Dr Neary removed the uteruses of young women in childbirth, so in these cases he deprived this group of women of their reproductive organs, sometimes the uterus but more frequently the ovaries . . . The commonest unnecessary procedure was that of bilateral salpingo-oophorectomy . . . In many cases they had private consultations with Dr Neary . . .

Endometriosis
Many women were coerced into having their ovaries (and sometimes their uterus) removed on the basis that they had endometriosis . . . This diagnosis can only be suspected until it is diagnosed visually. Thus most women underwent surgery misled into believing that the diagnosis was certain . . . In many of these cases there was in fact no endometriosis found by the pathologist . . . In fact, endometriosis is uncommonly so severe that it requires radical surgery . . . Many of the

women told us that they were informed by Dr Neary that surgery for endometriosis was essential because the endometriosis would damage them irreparably, and/or might become malignant and could cause their untimely death. None of that is of course true. It is always a self-limiting condition and always gets better at the menopause. It is never a pre-malignant condition.

Benign Disease (Cysts)

On other occasions Dr Neary removed one or both ovaries for benign disease . . . that required only limited surgery. Oophorectomy is very seldom required in these circumstances, particularly in women many years before their expected menopause, and was definitely not in these cases.

Life-saving Surgery

We were repeatedly told by these women that Dr Neary told them post-operatively that he had saved their lives. Dr Neary exaggerated the difficulty of the operation in many cases, possibly in order to justify the radical surgery he performed. These were . . . self-evidently untrue.

Blood Loss

In her report Judge Clark considered that one of the possible motives for Dr Neary's caesarean hysterectomies was his fear of blood loss. No such excuse can be offered in these cases . . . We believe that a fear of excessive blood loss cannot possibly explain his cavalier treatment of women's reproductive organs.

Consent

A patient who consents to an operation on the sole basis of a diagnosis that has not been confirmed by anything other than a clinical hunch is being misled and should be informed that the diagnosis remains uncertain. Without such information the consent cannot be held to be informed. However, in addition to this, many of the women in this group had no idea that their ovaries would be removed as part of their surgery or believed they would only be removed if there was ovarian pathology – a condition that was usually not met. A considerable number of these operations therefore lacked any proper consent.

The doctors concluded:

This visit uncovered a very large number of unnecessary operations on women's reproductive organs. No gynaecologist will in their career make universally correct judgements. However, the sheer number of operations in this sample of operations performed by a single surgeon indicates a major underlying issue.

Dr Neary appears not to have been a technically incompetent surgeon. Immediate surgical complications were not a feature here.

Dr Neary appears to have reached diagnoses, frequently incorrectly, based on clinical examination alone, and on that basis performed radical surgery, even though at operation it was clear that the diagnosis had been incorrect. Yet faced with the facts at the time of surgery he continued in very many cases to deprive women of their reproductive organs and their own sex hormones. In our view the recurrent nature of this behaviour, and the absence of evidence of inadequate surgical technique, raises very troubling questions about his motives.

Small wonder, then, that the women felt assaulted and mutilated.

Undoubtedly the greatest sadness for the group has been the refusal of the government and the Minister to stand by the promise given to named women to include them in some form of redress. There are approximately thirty-five excluded women in all. They all have strong medical reports from the same doctors who provided reports for the women who had unwarranted peripartum hysterectomies and oophorectomies. A full review of Neary's practices recommended in 2000 has never been conducted.

We believe that this exclusion, clear from the earliest days, was a direct result of the anxieties of the Departments of Health and Finance about opening "cans of worms" in this area of medical practice. They were furthermore determined to "ring-fence" the potential for redress to a very tight "egregious" form of damage to patients. Our long and protracted meetings with the Department and ministers, about the scope of the Lourdes Hospital Inquiry, were the result of our determination to include all damaged women into its scope and the equal determination by the government and officials that they wouldn't. Talks with Judge Harding

Clark, concerning eligibility for redress, were also unnecessarily drawn out because of these exclusions. Government used the Medical Council's findings as the lynchpin to which the inquiry should be attached lest "floodgates" be opened. Thus they have so far been able to exclude a very damaged and hurt number of women from the justice and validation they so badly need for recovery.

Why is redress important in healing? It is about people being able to forgive. It is about avoiding the need for retribution. It reunites the damaged person with others, it helps to mend the broken trust. This is especially true in medical negligence.

Because a hospital is a place of healing, because a doctor is a healer, damaged patients have terrible difficulty in getting their heads around the violation of trust, the deep injury to the soul. It damages the patient's way of looking at the world, their feeling of safety in it. But importantly, because redress makes forgiveness easier and removes the need for revenge, it helps everyone behave in an orderly way.

Redress is a marker, an apology, an acknowledgement, a making of amends. It is good for the community too because it means the people responsible are required to contribute and reflect on the damage. It requires people to change. It makes it much less likely it will happen again. So it is needed on many levels – personal, spiritual, political, and indeed medical.

Its spiritual dimension of acknowledgement, reparation and forgiveness allows a mending. That is why it is so important. That is a very important element of our group meetings. The re-establishment of that vital reconnection with others. These women have been excluded from this healing. Women who were three months, three weeks, or even three days over forty are excluded. So too were Orla and Sandra, whose babies died. They fought so hard for everyone else and they are denied healing for themselves.

The door cannot be closed on this terrible matter until they are included.

34

Why?

From the beginning people have asked about Neary: who was he and why did he do it?

Michael Neary was loved and respected by some and loathed by others. Many were afraid of his volatility, others excused it, some admired it. We know that someone even removed patient files from the hospital to help him. It is clear that he was very different things to different people, as the following comments from former patients and some colleagues show:

"I wouldn't be here today were it not for him."

"He had a butcher's touch about him."

"He was a good and caring doctor."

"Sneary Neary I called him."

"Always in the hospital."

"He had hands like shovels hurting you."

"He had a personality disorder."

As the story unfolded, everyone involved found great difficulty in coming to terms with what they found. What do his actions say about the man who was king of the maternity and gynaecology units of the Lourdes Hospital for so long?

We will never answer the "why" question fully. But we should opt for the most benign explanation consistent with the facts. This is the method we adopted in relation to Neary. This is important from the point of view of both the women and Neary. The women are done no service by attributing evil intent where there was none. On the other hand, refusing to see it where it clearly is a strong possibility is equally inappropriate.

The very first report, the IOG's Report, ruled out medical necessity as the reason for many of the caesarean hysterectomies Neary performed. The lack of direct sterilisation procedures and a fear of blood remained as possible explanations. But this review did not speak to the women. That they went into hospital to have their first, second or third baby and experience this wonder was not factored in. The women knew it was not sterilisation. Initially, they believed it was enormous blood loss that caused their own particular personal tragedy. There was no shortage of blood in the hospital for those who needed it. And in many cases it was not needed. But hysterectomies followed. The young age of the women and the low number of children they had made the sterilisation explanation unlikely. Judge Harding Clark firmly ruled out the shortage of blood and sterilisation explanations in her report.

She identified a phobic fear of blood and of losing a woman in childbirth as the most probable explanation for his extraordinary rate of caesarean hysterectomy. But Judge Harding Clark herself discovered a second pathology in Neary's practice, not explained by a fear of blood or death in childbirth. This was in his gynaecology practice: the large-scale and unnecessary removal of both ovaries in young women. This denied some women the right to have children and plunged them all into a very early menopause.

Why did he do this?

The Clements and Porter report, which exclusively dealt with the unnecessary removal of both ovaries in young and middle-aged women, ruled out a fear of blood as reason for this surgery. These were pre-planned operations which women were persuaded they needed for non-existent or benign disease. Clements and Porter had serious concerns about Neary's motivation for performing this surgery.

What do the women think?

Many women felt they owed their lives to Neary because he told them he rescued them from near catastrophe. He sometimes pointed to the cemetery, which could be seen from the ward, and told women they would be there now if it were not for his expertise. "You almost left here in a box"; "You were a nightmare case"; "I worked on you all night"; "You bled like a pig"; "You were one in a million" were common explanations given for the emergency hysterectomies. Judge Harding Clark too identified Neary's practice of poking at bleeding points, which may have caused problems for some women. But we know that excessive bleeding was not the cause in most cases, so Neary's habit of poking at bleeding points is difficult to understand. Some women believe he needed to be the centre of attention and that his heroics served this function for him. Everyone admired him, was grateful to him, considered him to be almost god-like in his skill. Some think of this as a form of Munchausen's syndrome.

Many women tell how Neary treated them physically and emotionally. He told many women he "removed the cradle and left the play pen" as a way of explaining a caesarean hysterectomy. Many feel that a hatred of women, or at least of the process of pregnancy and childbirth, explains this. Many too believe that he degraded them with his use of language in times of crisis in their lives. He told Rosemary Cunningham when she challenged him as to why he had removed her ovary that he did "not like her bloody ovary anyway". And then there was the terrible scar many of his patients were left with after a caesarean section. We know he was a good and competent surgeon. Why did he do this?

Some women and more of the men believe he is a sexual deviant and performed mutilating surgery on them "for fun". This explanation gained weight after the original consultation with Dr Roger Clements. He referred to Neary's behaviour as psychotic and to the wounds he inflicted as mutilation. Then, of course, there's Anne's story. The day following her caesarean hysterectomy, a doctor asked her if she had noticed "anything unpleasant while in theatre". She hadn't, but she thought this an extraordinary question. She didn't have bad memories but was disturbed by the question.

Neary refused to accept that he did anything wrong. The Medical Council regretted this "absence of insight and objectivity", given the huge statistical evidence Neary provided against himself.

The Council commented too on "the non-existence of any mechanism either within the hospital or elsewhere to ensure that such errors as occurred might be corrected or that a pattern of adverse or unusual outcomes should be properly monitored".

That brings us to the culture explanation – that in some way the culture in the hospital was responsible for this dreadful story. The women believe that the power of consultants in the hospital, the fear of them, the silence of the nuns, midwives and other professionals, the refusal to listen to the women themselves, allowed the scandal to continue unchecked for a very long time. But they do not believe it *caused* it to happen. For that, they point to Neary himself. A corrupt culture let him do what he did for twenty-five years. It did not make him remove their wombs and ovaries unnecessarily. Culture did not stop him.

"Ann", the midwife from Northern Ireland, stopped him. When explaining why, she wrote:

I have worked as a midwife since January 1994. I have always done my best to care for the women and their families in my care throughout my midwifery and nursing career. Faced with difficulties and challenges in the past, I relied upon my training and my personal supports to change the things that conflicted with that care ethos. I have an unshakeable belief in the rights of women and their families to receive the best maternal care at any one time. That was my only motive for my words and deeds of 1997 and 1998 in Drogheda in support of these families.

The corrupt culture didn't stop "Ann" doing what her ethos of care required of her. No more than it caused Neary to do as he did.

Two and a half years after the publication of the Lourdes Report, Dr Roger Clements invited Cathriona, Jim and me to London to speak to his colleagues about Neary. The story had gone quiet in Ireland since the recession descended and made all talk of appropriate redress for the remaining thirty-five women almost impossible. We were glad of the interest and support this visit provided.

It was hot and sunny in Harley Street on the afternoon of that early June day in 2009. Women in sun dresses and men in sunglasses, carried briefcases in this part of London. As we squeezed into the lift of this elegant London house, we talked of the young Irish women who came here to be told the truth.

As we drank tea and orange juice in his living room, I asked Roger Clements why Neary did these terrible things to Cathriona, to Nicola, to all the women – and still says he saved their lives.

"It is my opinion that Neary is a psychopath," he said, looking straight at us. "Jack the Ripper did hysterectomies but he had to kill the women first. Neary didn't. They were prostrate on an operating table for him. An obstetrician being afraid of blood is like a scaffolder being afraid of heights – give me a break. And there's no blood issue in the gynaecological cases. In the summer of 2000, when I was asked by Hugh – that's right, that's his name, isn't it?" Roger asked Cathriona.

"Yes, Hugh Thornton."

"Anyway, when I was asked by Hugh to see eleven women he thought had unnecessary caesarean hysterectomies, I didn't believe this was possible. I had seen patients of another obstetrician, Ledwith, in the past."

"The fastest gynaecologist in England," Cathriona interjected.

"That's right; about one in ten of those cases were problematic, so I thought, one or two of Neary's maybe, but not all eleven. But it was true. All eleven were unnecessary. What's happening to the criminal case?"

"Nothing," I said, "at the moment anyway."

"Why? What about our report, Dr Porter's and mine, the one we did after going to Dublin?"

"The DPP says it is not enough to prosecute him because it's too hard to prove intent. The women who complained to the guards underwent caesarean hysterectomies. None of the women who had both ovaries removed have complained yet. It's a very big thing for a woman; we need to go at their speed. Besides, they only know for a short while how unnecessary their operations were." Roger was not impressed. "It was castration, pure and simple."

"In Ireland we don't send Neary's sort to jail; we give them state pensions," Cathriona said.

Epilogue

It would be wonderful if there was a totally happy ending to this book, like a gift wrapped in pretty paper and tied with ribbons. That is not how it is.

Many questions still remain unanswered; in particular, the extent of the damage caused by Michael Neary to women over forty in the gynaecology ward of the Lourdes. This has never been systematically measured or quantified in any way. Neary himself has never accepted any responsibility for the harm he caused, maintaining that he saved the lives of the women.

A similar situation exists in relation to Michael Shine. His name was finally erased from the Medical Register on 24 November 2008. He was found guilty of professional misconduct in relation to three patients (teenage boys), on seven grounds, including assault/indecent assault (Medical Council Press release, 27 January 2009).

Neary's former patients believe some professionals have avoided engagement, responsibility and accountability. The people intimately involved in the initial handling of this scandal no longer work in the HSE. Dr Ambrose McLoughlin is now Registrar and CEO of the Pharmaceutical Society of Ireland. Jim Reilly is currently on secondment from the HSE. He works with Patient Focus, developing a much-needed patient advocacy service.

Professor Gerard Bury and later Dr John Hillery, during his Presidency of the Medical Council, continued to work for change. Dr Hillery made several public statements about the courage of the women and this was greatly appreciated. We found sympathy and admiration coming from both presidents.

The three doctors who exonerated Neary in 1998 underwent a Medical Council Fitness to Practise inquiry and were found guilty of professional misconduct in February 2007. While the FTP committee recommended sanctions, the Council decided to impose no sanctions, but the finding of misconduct was upheld. Prof. Prendiville and Dr Murphy sought judicial review of the lawfulness of these decisions. In December 2007, Judge Peter Kelly overturned the Council's decisions. He ruled that the Council had failed in its duty to conduct its disciplinary proceedings fairly. The finding against Dr Stuart was also reversed at a later date by the Council. Judge Kelly's ruling was not appealed by the Medical Council.

"Ann", the midwife, thankfully continues to practise her chosen profession in Ireland. Irish women have benefited greatly from her courage. Much-needed change has occurred as a direct result of her actions.

A statutory complaints system now exists in the HSE and nowadays patients regularly obtain access to their records – a far cry from the obstacles faced by the Neary patients. Audit and risk management processes are developing in most hospitals. However, it is undeveloped as yet and there is much room for improvement. The Health Information and Quality Authority has been established with its headquarters in Cork. It has conducted a number of far-reaching investigations since its establishment in 2007, including the inquiry into the delayed diagnosis of breast cancer patient Rebecca O'Malley in the Midwestern Regional Hospital in Limerick.

There is much need for a comprehensive national patient advocacy service so that all patients with anxieties about their care can receive an independent second opinion easily and cheaply.

Much change has occurred in how the Medical Council does its business too. This is the result of recent changes to legislation by the Minister for Health and Children, Mary Harney. Though it is too soon to say how this will work out in the coming years, it is certain that a massive cultural change has occurred under the new legislation. Today there are thirteen non-medical members out of twenty-five, though some are members of associated professions. Fitness to Practise committees must have a majority of lay members – quite different from what the women faced in 2000. A number of hearings have been held in public, too. Closed doors have definitely opened. How much and how wide only time will tell. However, the signs are good. Furthermore, doctors will now be required to demonstrate their competence to practise as a condition of remaining on the Medical Register.

As for the women and men involved in this scandal, most have recovered and are getting on with their lives. They will never forget, however. Some women sadly have not come to terms to what happened to them and need continuing support. All of the women and men involved will continue to deal with the loss of unborn children and, in the future, unborn grandchildren.

I will be eternally grateful for the experience of knowing them and walking this road with them over the last ten years. The men were often strong silent types who supported their women at every hand's turn. Dr Tony O'Sullivan was remarkable in his clear thinking and courage too. I know the women involved are very appreciative of the many long nights he spent in the Boyne Valley Hotel helping them.

I would like to thank my husband, Wilfie. His support was indeed heroic. I could not have done it without him. In addition, my three children, Dave, Katie and Aideen, were helpful in every possible way. Brian Langan of Poolbeg demonstrated impressive patience and professionalism and I would like to thank him too for this.

The women have had a docudrama made about their experiences. Siobhan Burke of Saffron Pictures in conjunction with the researcher Sheila Ahern prepared this award-winning drama. *Whistleblower* was funded and transmitted by RTÉ in 2008. The production was very well received by the women and their families.

As to whether this can ever happen again, sadly no one can be sure it can't. It is safe to say, however, that it is much less likely given the new safeguards that are currently developing. But the price of quality patient care is eternal vigilance, not undue trust and loyalty. That is one of the many lessons of this terrible story.

POOLBEG WISHES TO
THANK YOU

for buying a Poolbeg book and will give you
20% OFF (and free postage*)
on any book bought on our website
www.poolbeg.com

Select the book(s) you wish to buy
and click to checkout.

Then click on the 'Add a Coupon' button
(located under 'Checkout') and enter
this coupon code

CAUEA15165

(Not valid with any other offer!)

POOLBEG

POOLBEG

WHY NOT JOIN OUR MAILING LIST
@ www.poolbeg.com and get some
fantastic offers on Poolbeg books

*See website for details